Rewire,
Rework,
Reclaim

Dr Rajiv Mehta is a senior consultant psychiatrist and vice chairperson at the Institute of Psychiatry and Behavioural Sciences, Sir Ganga Ram Hospital, New Delhi. He is a professor of psychiatry at the Ganga Ram Institute for Postgraduate Medical Education and Research, and the director of the Indian Council for Journalism and Juvenile Research. For over two decades, he has been helping patients bring positive changes in their lives. His first book was on self-improvement, *Speak to Anyone, Easily* (Rupa Publications India, 2018). His views on current lifestyle problems and their solutions are regularly sought by leading media and corporate houses.

'There are many books that have been written on stress, but in this one, Dr Mehta, who is a brilliant psychiatrist, has put together all his experience and knowledge gathered over the last several years. Loaded with so many ways to help deal with daily stressors, this book deserves a special place in every household.'

Dr Sanjay Chugh, senior consultant psychiatrist

'Rewiring negative thought patterns, reworking your ways to deal with stress and reclaiming a worry-free life—this is the book by Dr Mehta. It is for anyone seeking to break free from the clutches of depression.'

Dr Kersi Chavda, senior consultant psychiatrist, P.D. Hinduja National Hospital and Sir H.N. Reliance Foundation Hospital

'Rajiv's book covers all aspects related to modern-day stressors and stress—detailing the consequences and approaches, which are both preventive as well as curative. A must-read to make present living stress-free.'

RJ Raunac, Red FM, New Delhi

'In a world where all of us are contantly striving to lead a stress-free life, Dr Rajiv Mehta's book will serve as a ready reckoner for many. Dr Mehta's experience as one of the most senior psychiatrists in the country clearly reflects in the book and I'm sure will help every reader.'

RJ Khurafati Nitin, Big FM, New Delhi

'Dr Mehta's book is loaded with practical suggestions towards minimizing anxiety and depression and living life to the fullest.'

RJ Ashish Sharma, Ishq FM, New Delhi

'Dr Rajiv Mehta's *Rewire, Rework, Reclaim: How to Manage Stress* serves as a beacon of hope amidst the tumult of modern life. With insightful precision, Dr Mehta not only diagnoses the root causes of stress but also offers pragmatic solutions. Through this compelling work, readers are not only equipped to navigate the complexities of stress but are also inspired to reclaim control over their well-being.'

Harpal Singh Sokhi, chef and restauranteur

Also by the author

Speak to Anyone, Easily

The Dos and Don'ts of Communication in Difficult Times (Kindle)

∞

Praise for *Speak to Anyone, Easily*

'Rajiv approaches the "Dos and Don'ts" of communication in a manner that has immediate resonance with the reader—and this hasn't been done as effectively in any book I've read before.'

Dr Sanjay Chugh, senior consultant psychiatrist

'An extraordinary and useful book... Rajiv's research on the damaging impact of the casual approach to communication is an eye-opener for everyone.'

Dr Anjali Chhabria, senior consultant psychiatrist
and author of *Death Is Not the Answer*

Rewire, Rework, Reclaim

How to
MANAGE STRESS

DR RAJIV MEHTA

Published by
Rupa Publications India Pvt. Ltd 2024
7/16, Ansari Road, Daryaganj
New Delhi 110002

Sales centres:
Bengaluru Chennai
Hyderabad Jaipur Kathmandu
Kolkata Mumbai Prayagraj

Copyright © Dr Rajiv Mehta 2024

The information provided in this book is designed to provide helpful information on the subjects discussed. This book is not meant to be used, nor should it be used, to diagnose or treat any medical condition.
While every effort has been made to verify the authenticity of the information contained in this book, it is not intended as a substitute for medical consultation with a physician. The publisher and the author are in no way liable for the use of the information contained in this book.

All rights reserved.
No part of this publication may be reproduced, transmitted, or stored in a retrieval system, in any form or by any means, electronic, mechanical, photocopying, recording or otherwise, without the prior permission of the publisher.

P-ISBN: 978-93-6156-190-0
E-ISBN: 978-93-6156-939-5

First impression 2024

10 9 8 7 6 5 4 3 2 1

The moral right of the author has been asserted.

Printed in India

This book is sold subject to the condition that it shall not, by way of trade or otherwise, be lent, resold, hired out, or otherwise circulated, without the publisher's prior consent, in any form of binding or cover other than that in which it is published.

*To the Almighty, my father the late S.P. Mehta,
and Guruji Shyam Sunder Sharma*

Contents

Introduction	11
1. The ABC of Stress	17
2. Finding the Middle Ground in Parenting	31
3. The Power of Pause	39
4. Bound Together, Forever	47
5. The Side Effects of Temptation	56
6. The Motherhood Experience	64
7. Pressure of Procreation	73
8. Forever Unbound	90
9. The Modern Family	99
10. Life after Loss	108
11. The Empty Nest Syndrome	117
12. Solo Parenting	124
13. Health Is the True Wealth	133
14. Money, Money, Money...	141
15. The Price of Prosperity	150
16. When the Going Gets Tough	159

17. The Lows of a High	168
18. Let's Talk about Sex and Sexuality	179
19. When Virtual Becomes Reality	190
Acknowledgements	200

Introduction

Some days ago, I was taken aback when I heard my six-year-old daughter tell her mother, 'Don't take any tension, ma, I will complete my homework on time.' Even a six-year-old could recognize stress! That is the extent to which terms like stress, anxiety and depression have become an inseparable part of our daily language and our lives.

Moreover, considering the way urban living is patterned nowadays, it is no exaggeration to say that stress is bound to affect everyone at some time or the other.

As a practising psychiatrist for over two decades, among the scores of patients that I have treated, depression and anxiety have been the most common ailments.

According to the World Health Organization (WHO), depression is the leading cause of ill health and disability in the world today; in fact, WHO cites a *Lancet* study that states that from 2005 to 2015, globally there was an increase of over 18 per cent and around 15 per cent in the cases of depression and anxiety disorders, respectively.[*]

Support structures, however, have been lagging in both professional and familial spheres. Also, prevailing stereotypes

---

*World Health Organization, *Depression and Other Common Mental Disorders: Global Health Estimates*, 2017, https://tinyurl.com/498sca6t. Accessed on 12 March 2024.

about such conditions—that any mental health condition is 'madness' or denotes self-weakness—and the social stigma attached to them prevent many from seeing depression as just an ailment, and from seeking treatment that would enable them to lead a healthy, purposeful existence. A lack of awareness also prevents many from seeking help.

Those who do share their suffering invariably mention two things:

- the behavioural changes they see in themselves (which are termed 'stress'); and
- the reasons for those changes (which are termed 'stressors').

Generally, when people approach professionals, they talk more about the reasons that they think are responsible for the changes they are going through. However, the behavioural changes are the symptoms. They are quite similar across most people and are descriptive of disorders known as depression and anxiety.

Often, there is a tendency to use the terms stress, depression and anxiety interchangeably. But there are differences.

- Stress is the body's response to any demand for change caused by and with the aim of adjusting to pressure. It denotes the physical, emotional and behavioural changes that occur while dealing with the challenges that a person is confronted with. When stress is prolonged and severe enough that it impacts a person's social life, occupational life, or both, it becomes clinically significant enough to start intervention or treatment.
- Anxiety is a disorder marked by worries and apprehensions.

- Depression is a condition predominated by sadness.

Both depression and anxiety often coexist.

The Challenges of Our Present-Day Lives

Each person is required to fulfil many roles—they are a child, sibling, friend, spouse and partner; they are also an individual, student, employee and employer. Every role has aspects that can be seen as either advantageous or posing a problem—these problems are what we call stressors or stress triggers. Stressors can also be changes in external circumstances, such as job loss or illness in the family. Any life alteration requires continuous adjustments, which, when beyond one's coping abilities, can give rise to depressive and anxiety symptoms.

Based on my experience, I can say that these problems/stressors can be classified into general categories. While some of these have been part of humankind's existence for a long time, some have manifested with the increasing pace of urbanization and modern-day living—for instance, the demands placed on individuals in nuclear family set-ups to perform multiple roles that were earlier distributed across a joint family structure. The pressures have increased further with the pervasive presence of technology in our lives, to the extent that it almost seems to dominate our existence in every sphere.

There is a general perception that problems arising from a demanding lifestyle are bound to cause stress. In reality, all individuals facing such problems may not experience suffering. This raises several questions:

- Why are some more prone to suffering than others?

- Are the reasons for this genetic, or does resilience in personality depend more on a person's conscious lifestyle choices?
- Does the difference in dealing with stressors decide whether stress will lead to depression/anxiety or not?
- How does one deal with these commonly occurring situations in life to protect oneself from falling into depression?

As a responsible member of society and a long-time mental health professional, I have often felt the need to share my insights on stress and stressors, anxiety and depression. The inflection point came in the form of Covid-19, the pandemic that hit India in early 2020, bringing with it an unfamiliar protocol for survival—initially, a stringent nationwide lockdown at the end of March 2020, and thereafter an extended period of 'social isolation', which involved being confined to and working from home.

On the one hand, the severe restriction of movement and activities brought on by the idea of 'social isolation' led to terrible economic losses as businesses folded up and a large section of society found itself bereft of jobs. Being housebound for long periods in such conditions led to a rise in instances of domestic violence and child abuse.[*] There were many cases of persons taking their lives as well.

On the other hand, the media started reporting an

---

[*]Ghoshal, Rakhi, 'Twin Public Health Emergencies: Covid-19 and Domestic Violence', *Indian Journal of Medical Ethics*, Vol. 5, No. 3, 2020, pp. 195–9, https://tinyurl.com/57z6xrea. Accessed on 12 March 2024; Pallansch, Jennifer, et al., 'Intimate Partner Violence, Sexual Assault, and Child Abuse Resource Utilization During Covid-19', *Western Journal of Emergency Medicine*, Vol. 23, No. 4, 2022, pp. 589–96, https://tinyurl.com/4uxc2xd5. Accessed on 12 March 2024.

alarming spike in stress, depression and anxiety across all age groups and sections of society.* Webinars focussing on the three were conducted with a sense of urgency.** The importance of mental health issues was discussed widely.

This juncture was an important milestone as it signalled a recognition of the need for mental well-being as a significant factor affecting the quality of life.

My life, too, underwent a change during the pandemic. The almost-frenzied routine of home, hospital and clinic was paused for a while. For the first time in years, I had some time on my hands. What better use of it than to pen down the learnings of my practice to help people recognize the symptoms of stress and how to manage themselves, thereby helping them rise above their suffering? Finally, my long-standing dream has been realized.

I have tried to provide an introduction to the topic of stress—its definition, biology, impacts and association with major medical diseases; the measurement of the intensity of stress; and finally, some of the techniques that can help a person protect herself from or handle stress.

Every person has their own way of thinking. When encountering a new situation fraught with problems, thinking along predictable lines may not help them avoid stress. What is needed is an alternate view from a well-wisher or a mental health professional who sees what the person facing

---

*Covid-19 Pandemic Triggers 25% Increase in Prevalence of Anxiety and Depression Worldwide', *World Health Organization*, 2 March 2022, https://tinyurl.com/ytvt556. Accessed on 12 March 2024.

**The author and his colleagues received a high volume of webinar requests from media and corporate entities, leading to an unprecedented frequency of webinars.

the problem is unable to see, and provides a solution in the form of medication and psychotherapy.

This book aims to serve the purpose of such a well-wisher. It is based on my experiences with countless patients and describes the common stressors and their consequences that the current generation faces, and indicates ways in which this generation can handle the ever-increasing presence and impacts of stress before it increases to an extent that it requires medical intervention.

The fact that stress is an epidemic of epic proportions needs to be realized, for it can play a vital role in indicating a predisposition to, or in the precipitation and perpetuation of, various mental and physical illnesses. If not treated, affected individuals find it hard to lead a productive personal and professional life.

regulatory capacity of an organism'.[2] Put simply, it is the reaction a person shows when placed under excessive pressures or demands. Here, 'excessive' has a specific meaning—more than the individual is capable of handling. The capacity to handle excessive pressure varies from person to person.

Pressure that is not excessive for a person at one point can become so later, as the coping ability varies over time depending on several factors—the frequency of and familiarity with pressures in the past, the difference in age, and the availability of social and financial support.

Importantly, the perception of a given event or situation determines how much stress is felt. An event seen as mildly challenging would probably lead to less stress; if it is perceived as threatening, or overwhelming, the stress felt would be much higher. For instance, waiting for a cab to go to a wedding may not trigger as much stress as waiting for a cab when you're running late for a flight.

If a less-threatening pressure, or stressor, elicits an intense response that impacts socio-occupational life, it is an overreaction and calls for an intervention.

Getting the Terms Right

Many make the common mistake of using the terms stressor/stress trigger and stress interchangeably. A stressor is the actual or perceived event, whereas stress is the individual's emotional and physical response to it.

---

[2]Koolhaas, Jaap M., et al., 'Stress Revisited: A Critical Evaluation of the Stress Concept', *Neuroscience & Biobehavioral Reviews*, Vol. 35, No. 5, 2011, pp. 1291–301, https://tinyurl.com/yh9nw6s2. Accessed on 12 March 2024.

1

The ABC of Stress

Why Are You So Stressed?

'Being stressed' is a phrase that has entered our daily vocabulary and existence. For individuals confronted with a rapidly altering and challenging environment, as is characteristic of our times, stress is very common. It has become a phenomenon seen across all age groups.

The word 'stress' comes from the Latin word *stringere*, which means 'to draw tight'. The term, or the condition it denotes, is less than 100 years old; it was in the 1930s–40s that the Hungarian–Canadian endocrinologist Hans Selye developed the stress theory, exploring the effects of stress on the human body.[1]

Stress, like happiness, isn't easy to define. In their review study on stress in 2011, Koolhaas described it as a condition in which 'an environmental demand exceeds the natural

---

[1]Viner, Russell, 'Putting Stress in Life: Hans Selye and the Making of Stress Theory', *Social Studies of Science*, Vol. 29, No. 3, 1999, pp. 391–410, https://tinyurl.com/2w26fhry. Accessed on 13 March 2024.

The simple ABC stress model (A+B=C) created by the well-known American psychologist Albert Ellis explains this well.[3] He posits that:

A = activating event, namely the stressor
B = beliefs, thoughts or perceptions about A
C = emotional, physical and behavioural consequence/reaction, or stress

Even events perceived as positive, such as marriage or promotion, can be stressors for many, for they demand adjustment to a new situation.

Stressors and stress are of two kinds—they can be acute and short-lived, or chronic and long-lasting. A stressor that impacts one only for a short duration can be handled. The body and mind react and generally recover soon to return to their pre-stress, more relaxed state.

Chronic stress, like chronic illness, is altogether different. Continuous exposure to stressor(s), without enough recovery time for the body and mind to adjust, often leads to chronic stress. This type of stress is long-lasting. It can give rise to brain disorders, most commonly depression and anxiety, which require treatment.

Good Stress versus Bad Stress

Stress is bad when it is continuous and beyond an individual's coping ability, leading to it impacting one's life. But there are times when stress can be good, too. In fact, in

---

[3]Selva, Joaquín, 'What Is Albert Ellis' ABC Model in CBT Theory?', *PositivePsychology.com*, 8 March 2018, https://tinyurl.com/msw93tw3. Accessed on 12 March 2024.

the words of Hans Selye, 'Stress is the spice of life.'[4]

When a short-term stressor is well within a person's coping ability and leads to a positive reaction, it is called good stress, or eustress—for instance, the nervousness experienced before exams can actually improve one's performance. On the other hand, stress that starts from the first day of classes and lingers on, creating negative consequences such as a sharp dip in a student's learning capacity and inferior grades, is called bad stress, or distress.

Good and bad stress should be seen as a continuum. There is a fine line between the two, and it varies from person to person. Workaholics who say they do their best under pressure thrive on stress. It is satisfying and rewarding for them. They get stressed when they have nothing to do. However, when stress becomes chronic, it can be damaging for them, too.

The experience of stress depends on multiple factors such as one's biological make-up, perception of stress, the intensity, number and duration of stressors, and stress management and coping skills. For all practical purposes, the stress that is being discussed in this book is distress.

Stress and Its Relationship with the Brain

When we experience any kind of pressure, our brain assesses it. Then it starts mobilizing its resources. The sympathetic nervous system automatically prepares the body for action (fighting or fleeing) by activating the

---

[4]Selye, Hans, 'A Personal Message from Hans Selye', *Journal of Extension*, 1980, pp. 6–11, https://tinyurl.com/ymazfu8h. Accessed on 12 March 2024.

hypothalamic–pituitary–adrenal axis, namely the brain's 'stress circuit', which is responsible for maintaining the body's balance through the regulation of vital functions like the digestive system, the immune system, moods, and the body's energy levels. Once the pressure recedes, the parasympathetic nervous system takes over and restores normalcy.

In today's times, the increasing presence of chronic and numerous stressors makes this balancing act difficult and complicated. The body and brain don't always get it right.

Under excessive stress, there is an alteration in the activity of the brain's nerve cells in order to manage the increased demand on the body's various systems to deal with the pressure. This leads to various structural and chemical changes in the brain. It is this overload that gets expressed behaviourally as depression, anxiety and other mental health problems.

Wherever possible, it is advisable to act immediately when you become aware of a stressor. Better still, learn stress management techniques as a preventative measure, a way of life. For, once a stressor leads to severe consequences, professional intervention in the form of medication and psychotherapy becomes necessary. Lifestyle changes by themselves may help in milder forms of illness.

It is important to remember that medication is not an indication of a person's weakness or weak resolve. All it means is that the brain system has suffered damage at a microscopic level, and requires help to repair itself. In the absence of treatment, problems can get aggravated, leading to multi-system consequences. Here, medicines fulfil a need; they do not spell dependency.

Signs and Symptoms of Stress

Multiple signs of acute, short-lived stress manifest as the body pumps in adrenaline, the 'fight or flight' chemical. There are changes at three levels—physical (bodily), emotional and behavioural—which are enumerated below.

In the early days of humankind, stress was nature's way of ensuring survival potential. The physical changes experienced are similar to those brought upon by emergencies perceived as life-threatening: the heart rate and blood pressure increase, sending more blood to the muscles and lungs; the muscles tense up, ready for action; breathing becomes rapid to increase the supply of air; and the pupils dilate for better visibility.

Emotionally, people can feel anxious, angry, frustrated, overwhelmed and fearful. It can cause an individual to overreact or under-react; annoyance becomes anger; and concern turns into anxiety. Sometimes it also leads to withdrawal, avoidance and giving up quickly. These are symptoms of distress.

These responses, which were appropriate for primitive survival, are inappropriate in non-life-threatening situations, such as misplacing a key or failing a driving test.

The symptoms of chronic stress are those of depression and anxiety disorders, which can range from mild to severe, and may change in severity depending on the duration and number of stressors.

Depression denotes a dip in mood, energy, pleasure, enjoyment, confidence, concentration, motivation, decision-making abilities, sense of humour, appetite, sleep, libido, self-worth, hope and willingness to live. On rare occasions, some people may exhibit binge eating or increased sleep and libido.

Anxiety or panic attacks are characterized by blurred or double vision, a dry mouth and throat, difficulty swallowing, shallow and rapid breathing, palpitations, nausea and vomiting, excessive sweating, cold extremities, goosebumps, tremors, frequent urination or defecation, nervousness, and nail-biting, fidgeting, hair-twirling or hair-pulling. There are worries and apprehensions, ruminations on a single thought, and undue fear. All this leads to lowered productivity, absenteeism, difficulty in relationships, and sometimes suicide.

How Constant Stress Impacts Various Body Systems

The brain, which activates its nerve cells to react to pressure, is the master switchboard of the body, controlling other organs. No wonder that eventually every body system is affected by stress—it happens earlier on for some, later for others; the effect is minimal for some, major for others. However, no organ is spared from the impact of chronic stress.

Stress can predispose one to, and precipitate and exacerbate the symptoms of, a wide variety of disorders. It is associated with five leading causes of death: heart ailments, cancer, lung diseases, accidents and suicides.

Stress impacts body systems in various ways:

- Pain in the neck (and other places): The muscles contract and become tense under stress, resulting in pain in the region of the head, neck and lower back. This may lead to muscle spasms and cramping, grinding of teeth (bruxism) and calf pain.

- Taking stress to heart: The elevation of adrenaline levels during stress increases heart rate and blood pressure, causes constriction of blood vessels and increases the rate of blood clotting, thereby increasing proneness to heart diseases. Research shows a disturbing rise in heart ailments among the younger generations.[5] It is becoming quite common to hear about heart attacks suffered by young adults who are too stressed.
- Inability to digest stress: The gastrointestinal tract is a favoured site for the accumulation of stress. Stress impacts the secretion of digestive juices and the gastrointestinal tract's motility. Gas, acidity, belching, constipation and weight loss/gain are common stress-related complaints. It also contributes to gastroesophageal reflux disease (GERD), irritable bowel syndrome (IBS), colitis and Crohn's disease.
- Fatal sugar cravings: Under stress, the body requires more glucose for physical action, and the brain requires it for quickening the thinking process. Chronic stress leads to chronic sugar cravings, which increases the chances of diabetes, obesity and higher cholesterol levels, as well as their related consequences.
- Compromised immune system: Chronic stress weakens the immune system, leading to decreased resistance to bacteria, viruses and allergens. The

---

[5] Sun Jiahong, et al., 'Global, Regional, and National Burden of Cardiovascular Diseases in Youths and Young Adults Aged 15–39 Years in 204 Countries/Territories, 1990–2019: A Systematic Analysis of Global Burden of Disease Study 2019', *BMC Medicine*, Vol. 21, 2023, https://tinyurl.com/29fyxcty. Accessed on 12 March 2024.

likelihood of cold, flu and allergies increases with stress.
- Loss of libido: Stress negatively impacts the libido of both men and women. It can reduce and even eliminate the pleasure of physical intimacy. This could lead to marital discord and be a reason for separation or divorce. Stress significantly accounts for infertility problems.
- Change in weight: Stress can lead to either weight loss or gain. Preoccupation with the pressure at hand can lead to a decrease in appetite and loss of taste, too. Some, however, experience cravings for sweet and fried foods during anxiety. Overeating or binge eating may act as a distraction from distress, eventually leading to weight gain.

Cancers and various skin conditions like psoriasis and lupus are also linked to stress.

The Impact of Stress on Relationships

Stress makes a person irritable or withdrawn, or both. Friends and family may not understand what is going on, or why the person is stressed despite their best intentions and support. Eventually they may become stressed themselves, thus escalating the cycle, which could lead to further distress.

How Stressed Are You?

Aids can be used to objectively measure and interpret stress levels:

- Stress gauge: Draw a line and mark on it a scale from 0 (no stress) to 10 (extreme stress). Subjectively assess

the stress and give yourself a score on the scale. This is a simple method to measure stress levels, and can be used on a daily basis or as per need. Being visual, it is convenient and can help you compare the changes in your scores easily.
- Stress journal: Maintain a record of problems encountered. The stressor and the stress level can be noted in a tabular format, thus identifying either or both the acute and chronic pressures and reactions. It acts as a cue for when to use stress-management techniques and also helps in planning the next move/day accordingly.
- The stress-symptom scale: A questionnaire, it is an objective measure of stress levels, which can also measure cumulative stress and assess the impact of stress-management techniques. Some freely available scales are the Perceived Stress Scale,[6] the Perceived Stress Questionnaire[7] and the DASS.[8]

Managing Stress

Stress can be managed through a three-pronged approach that involves:

---

[6] Metcalf, Michael, 'The Perceived Stress Scale: Measure How Stressed You Are', *marlee,* https://tinyurl.com/2ys4kujx. Accessed on 29 April 2024.

[7] Levenstein, Susan, et al., 'Development of the Perceived Stress Questionnaire: A New Tool for Psychosomatic Research', *Journal of Psychosomatic Research*, Vol. 37, No. 1, 1993, pp. 19–32, https://tinyurl.com/3t4vj6kx. Accessed on 12 March 2024.

[8] *Depression Anxiety Stress Scales (DASS)*, 18 August 2023, https://tinyurl.com/5cupfx2d. Accessed on 12 March 2024.

- managing the stressors;
- changing the thought process; and
- managing the stress response.

The techniques can be general or stressor-specific.

- Managing stressors: Stress triggers can range from something seemingly minor, like a broken shoelace on a crowded metro, to something dramatic, like a divorce or a serious illness. The number of potential stressors is endless.

    By altering, minimizing or eliminating potential stressors, one can save oneself from stress. For instance, by taking a few minutes to put things in their place, one can prevent the irritability that the sight of a cluttered home triggers, or by spending consciously, one can save oneself from the stress of high credit-card bills. Mastering problem-solving and time-management skills is vital.

- Changing the thought process: A person's beliefs, thoughts, perceptions and interpretations are critical for determining how much stress they feel. When a situation or stress trigger cannot be changed—say, during a divorce or while pursuing work targets—the perception of the stressor needs to be altered. It's not the situation itself but the perception of it that governs stress. One's perception determines whether a situation feels overwhelming or capable of being controlled. With experience and feedback, one can learn to see things differently. For instance, for a person waiting in a long queue, two different ways of thinking—'I hate waiting' as opposed to 'let me use this time and organize my work-list'—will make all the difference in stress levels.

- Managing stress responses: Even if a stressor cannot be undone and one's mindset remains unchanged, mastering stress-relieving techniques to relax the body and calm the mind is useful.

Common Solutions

Here are some everyday solutions you can use to prevent yourself from succumbing to the unhealthy impacts of stress:

- Socializing with relatives and friends can help you air emotions and view problems differently. It is a well-known fact that pursuing social relationships is associated with a healthier and longer life.
- It is important to express the need for help from friends and family when you feel you are unable to manage the situation. Won't you help them in their time of need? No one is born with a comprehensive set of abilities. After all, the editor's experience has helped shape my writing.
- Being assertive or open about your views in a relationship, without giving in to anger or guilt, helps. Both extreme passivity and aggressiveness are harmful to the self and others. Assertive behaviour, which occupies the middle ground between passivity and aggressiveness, helps create a defined interpersonal boundary and a stress-free life. One needs to repeatedly practise it to learn its finer nuances.
- To introspect on your life—enjoying achievements, pondering mistakes, revising the ways you work or maintain relationships—is important for your development and can help you face difficulties as well.

- Having clear principles (values according to which you organize your life) and priorities (deciding what your real needs are as opposed to luxuries) is worthwhile, for this reduces your chances of being exploited or manipulated. Knowing your strengths and weaknesses, and finalizing needs and goals according to your abilities, principles and desires help you lead a satisfying life.
- Being organized ensures that stress is kept at bay. In today's fast-paced world, if certain aspects of life like personal documentation, finances and time are well organized, stress remains at a distance. Time management should include time for work, family, recreation and vacations. Financial organization should include saving for health and emergencies.
- Exercise is the best antidepressant and is also the least utilized. Exercise—intense physical exercise done regularly for a minimum of half an hour per day—increases the supply of endorphins (happy hormones) in the brain, creating a bulwark against stress. Besides, exercise boosts one's confidence and offers an opportunity to make friends through outdoor group activities.
- Relaxation exercises work on the idea that relaxation and stress are opposites, and hence can't coexist. Jacobson's progressive muscle relaxation (JPMR) is an easy technique.
- Yoga and meditation help in calming the mind.
- Today, there are many ways available to keep stress at bay. People can choose anything among diet therapy, pet therapy, aromatherapy, music therapy, humour, visualization, hypnosis, spiritualism and altruism.

Our lives today, particularly in metros and cities, are such that they create frequent stress triggers. To be aware of these triggers and actively pursue approaches to minimize their presence in our lives is not only possible but essential if we want to lead a healthy, fulfilling life.

2

Finding the Middle Ground in Parenting

According to Darwin's Origin of Species, *it is not the most intellectual of the species that survives; it is not the strongest that survives; but the species that survives is the one that is able best to adapt and adjust to the changing environment in which it finds itself.*

—Leon C. Megginson[9]

That adaptation, or adjustment, is essential for survival is exemplified by the evolution of humankind, having outlasted mightier creatures that roamed the earth once only to face extinction.

Someone might say adjustment or adaptation was required in the past but not now, for the world is a different place. They would be wrong because adjustment is needed

---

[9]Megginson, Leon C., 'Lessons from Europe for American Business', *The Southwestern Social Science Quarterly*, Vol. 44, No. 1, 1963, pp. 3–13, https://tinyurl.com/c89425u2. Accessed on 12 March 2024.

when one is confronted with a difficult situation. It involves both intelligence and strength—intelligence to know that change is required and the strength to bring about that change. These experiences, and their lessons, get absorbed to be applied in similar situations in life in the future.

But what happens when a person who has never faced any obstacle, who has had everything for the asking, faces a trying situation?

A person who has not faced any hurdles in life is less likely to develop the coping skills required to face the challenges that arise in life, for ambitions and obstacles are what forge a resilient personality.

Picture this backdrop to the life of a middle-class family in present times: the age of aspirational consumerism is firmly in place. The joint family system has given way to a nuclear family set-up. Also, the number of children per family has declined, whereas per capita incomes have risen. Products that were considered a luxury are now available to all—dropped at the doorstep, to be returned or replaced if not liked.

Now, picture the scenes from the life of a middle-class family unfold in this consumerist 'paradise'. Today's parents:

- don't wish to subject their child to any kind of pain
- give their child whatever is demanded, out of love or guilt
- think, 'Why are we earning if we don't fulfil our child's desires?'
- meet the child's every demand even if it is beyond their capacity, despite realizing that fulfilling the demand would create more problems

Pampering is the current parenting trend; it starts at a very early age, when children are showered with numerous gifts. Working parents feel guilty and frustrated that they are unable to give quality time to their children, hence they try to compensate through gifts and by agreeing to whatever the child demands. Materialism becomes the answer to the parents' sense of guilt and the child's emotional needs, which is definitely not the way to nurture children. Nothing can replace the time a parent can devote to the child.

Sometimes, the child emotionally blackmails the parents by throwing tantrums. Already burdened by too many responsibilities, the parents cave in. Their emotions override their reasoning, and the child gets their way. More importantly, children learn how to get their way through emotional blackmail, which spills into other relationships in their childhood and in the future. That is not a healthy way to begin and maintain friendships and relationships, for it is important to understand the other's viewpoint as well. Therefore, establishing boundaries and limitations by strongly and consistently standing up to children's tantrums is necessary.

Besides, one of the vital aspects of bringing up children is to teach them how to handle rejection and the disappointment of not getting something. Otherwise, their lives stand the risk of being marred with discontentment at every step. In fact, parents, too, need to understand where to draw the line by comprehending what is a necessity and what is a luxury for the child. Children eventually understand and learn to respect boundaries.

Impact of Pampering Children

If children are protected from having to face even the slightest of challenges, there is a direct impact on their ability to develop coping strategies. Deficient coping skills in children are sure to generate stress when they start facing real-life issues. And then depressive symptoms start surfacing. As life's challenges rise, so do depressive symptoms.

It is important to emphasize that for children, the idea that everything is available upon their asking imprints a subconscious message of abundance in their minds, and prevents them from realizing the true nature of their demands.

They develop unrealistic expectations from others. As adults, they are expected to understand that all their demands can't be met, especially immediately. But how will they demonstrate the patience that has not been cultivated at all till then?

Unmet needs give rise to frustration that may develop into a painful acknowledgement of self-deficiency. This creates confusion in the mind: 'Have I been wrong all along while my demands were being fulfilled, or is it only now that things have started going wrong?' This frustration, whether turned inwards or outwards, creates havoc in life. Eventually, the lives of everyone connected are severely impacted, and so is society.

Someone who has always been pampered generally expects the same treatment from everybody—friends, lovers, spouse and colleagues. But not everyone will understand the person's background and upbringing. Moreover, as an adult, the person is expected to overcome old habits by acquiring newer ones. What happens is that for such people it becomes difficult to establish, manage and maintain meaningful relationships outside the secure boundary of home, as they lack the ability to make a conscious effort to adjust. They may end up being loners.

Also, a lack of obstacles leads to either lack of ambition or lack of calibre. When a gulf develops between abilities and desires, anxiety starts to build up, more so when one's achievements are compared with those of their peers.

On the other hand, when children are brought up in an environment where love and care go hand in hand with enabling them to face challenges and responsibilities, they develop a well-adjusted personality, which gets a positive boost when they are able to handle tough situations. As adults, they are ready to take risks, which is necessary to be an achiever.

A person who has had a childhood of being pampered and cosseted will be prone to suffering stress, frustration, irritability, confusion, anxiety and depression when adversity rears its head, be it a career matter, a case of adjustment with friends or spouse, relocating to another city, or situations of increased responsibility such as a family member's illness. Any discrepancy between aptitude and attitude generates feelings of inadequacy and annoyance. Self-realization of limitations can lead to frustration, rebellion and depression in the long run. Some may veer towards dependence on drugs.

Parents also suffer, especially those whose life has just one focus—their children. They label it as their sacrifice. Unable to make personal, social or professional progress, it further pinches them when their child doesn't develop a well-balanced personality. The frustration may ultimately manifest as some kind of physical or mental illness.

Preparing Children to Face Life

First of all, adults need to learn the skill of balanced parenting. They need to realize that anything in excess is poison, be it rewards (demands met) or punishments.

Second, children should be routinely given their share of age-appropriate responsibilities, which in turn helps them develop coping skills. They need to know that rights and responsibilities go hand in hand. Their efforts should be positively reinforced by acknowledgement. Even if a family is in the position to provide all manner of worldly resources for the children, the development of a sense of responsibility is a must to enable them to become able individuals. That includes teaching them the value of money and how to handle it. It is the overall development of personality that puts a person on the path of achievement in life.

There is one more aspect regarding which the new generation needs to be grounded. 'Live like there's no tomorrow' is the credo of our consumerist society. Since the present-day wisdom about economic growth is centred on more consumption, this message is conveyed to the young from every quarter possible. Credit cards are waved around as wands that will help one buy anything one wants without the slightest pain (payments are always in the distant future so as to make them vanish). The lure of doorstep delivery through online shopping makes everything so easy.

Spending is primarily determined by the level of disposable income, which is definitely rising for present-day youth. Living it up, sometimes spending more than what is earned by taking loans and becoming members of the EMI economy, is common. The emphasis is on having all the comforts that are touted as essential for an upwardly mobile modern-day lifestyle in order to 'keep up with the Joneses', as the saying goes. The much publicized lifestyles of celebrities are also an influence.

This mindset of the present-day generation is supported by a general optimism that they can control every situation. Permanent income, expectations of future income and total wealth also influence their spending. On the flip side is the lack of savings, which often makes itself apparent during a crisis. Then, all at once, the modern lifestyle starts seeming fragile.

Often, to justify their lifestyles, people mention that some of the greatest philosophers have also said one must live in the present. However, what the philosophers meant was that neither should we be prisoners to our past, nor should we worry about the future. We should live in the present with a sense of purpose.

The question is, what does it mean to live with a sense of purpose in our times, as responsible human beings and as members of a family, community and humanity (particularly with crises like climate change coming to a head)? The first requirement would be to exercise self-control, change one's priorities, and reduce consumption. There is a need to prepare for contingencies, so savings are important. A balance between present and future needs, with an eye on the bigger picture, is what is required for a life as free of stress as possible.

In these times, when almost everything is monetized, stress and anxiety caused by unplanned expenses, such as during a health crisis, are most common. It is at such times that the bubble of comfort promised by credit cards and 'easy' loans breaks. This leads to intense stress, anxiety and, in some cases, suicide.

This is not to suggest that one must cling to the old. Every situation brings with it a new set of challenges, but what is essential is a grounded worldview based on distinguishing needs and basics from excessive comfort and consumption, and the foresight to plan for contingencies. In the present times of environmental crisis, for example, many of us can try to live by the rule of repairing rather than replacing things, to the greatest extent possible.

All of us need to relearn the lesson that there is beauty in a life of moderation. That does not mean living in a miserly fashion; it means living in a judicious manner.

3

The Power of Pause

Scenes from a typical day in a middle-class nuclear family in urban India: the working couple (or one partner) comes home close to dinner time. Then it's time for the gadgets—smartphone and television—to take over. Soon enough, it's bedtime.

The following morning, the children are off to school and the elders to their office. The time spent with oneself or the family is next to nothing. As for weekends, they are consumed by household errands. Before you know it, your life slips through your fingers like sand. All you know is that you have been busy.

Being busy is a relatively new phenomenon for humankind. Three or four decades ago, when the joint family was not entirely a thing of the past, in an economy that had not yet opened up, a nine-to-five job was the norm. There were less needs and demands, and less information about the world of never-ending 'choice' that an open economy promised.

Overall, responsibilities were divided among various members in the joint family. What people had was time— time to sit in the sun and gossip or read, time to visit friends and relatives, time to sleep.

As people switched gears to keep up with changing times, especially in cities, nuclear families became the norm, the focus turned on achievements, and material success became the yardstick for achievement and happiness. People started spending far more time travelling to and from work, for it was seen as the only way to forge ahead in life. Busyness became the norm, an accepted way of life.

Busyness Is Trending

Being busy is a quality much sought after. A person who is busy must be very important, and thus worth admiring, is the prevalent thinking in our times. Evaluating one's self-worth in comparison to others and the desire to be noticed and have power have become important goals of contemporary life. Constant action and being constantly connected are thought to be symbols of security, success and status. A person who is always on the go, whose every second and minute is accounted for, who has professional targets lined up and the drive to achieve them is considered to be worth emulating. This is the persona of success in our times.

If you ask professionals, they will say this is the only way to get ahead in life. Desiring a higher pay cheque involves changing jobs regularly and proving yourself all over again. Entrepreneurs are busy attending to their business as they plan for expansion. Life is dominated by work; work–life balance is skewed in urban India, especially for those in a corporate working environment.

Consequently, one's profession becomes the primary and, more often, only identity. In reality, an entrepreneur is also a spouse, parent, child, sibling, friend and a member of the community; these are the roles that lose out to busyness.

Regarding the women of the household, it is a different story. Whether they are working professionals or homemakers, they are burdened with multiple responsibilities that take up all their time. That is what society expects of them. New mothers sacrifice their independence to get fully involved in their children's rearing. Raising children, a full-time task, is seen to be their primary and only responsibility.

As for the children, they are kept busy with studies and extracurricular activities (which bring them the credits they need to enter a good university). If they like playing a sport, their parents put them in sports academies with the hope that their child might be the next prodigy, thus organizing their time to seconds and preventing the child from enjoying the game called life.

The question is, is being busy the same as being productive? Being busy denotes the amount of time spent doing something, while being productive is indicative of a proper utilization of time.

Then follows another question—at what cost to ourselves are we prioritizing busyness? Sometimes, even after realizing how futile and destructive constant busyness can be, people seem powerless to push the pause button. The act of being in a busy frame of mind burdens the brain, and prevents a person from partaking in the simple pleasures of life that keep a person on an even keel.

Impacts of Being Busy

There are several reasons why being excessively busy is not a very positive thing. Anything in excess is poisonous. Further, an excessive, obsessive pursuit of materialistic achievements to the exclusion of everything else can eventually lead to deep frustration.

It is important to recognize the dichotomy between material progress, which comes with its attendant frustrations, and happiness. In fact, it is during the course of the journey that happiness is experienced, not at the end of it.

Generally, the quests for material progress and happiness start together. For some time, they keep pace with each other. But with time, material progress gains primacy, for the idea of status is linked to it. The gap between material advancement and happiness keeps growing wider. Even in a limited sense, there's no time to savour an accomplishment as the next target looms ahead. Sooner or later, the idea of happiness is lost in the busyness of material growth.

The biggest loser in all this is the self. There's no time for the self. People often confuse 'me-time' with 'self-time'. The time spent in solitude in the pursuit of one's favourite activity or recreation is 'me-time'—it provides short-term happiness, mainly to the person involved. The time spent introspecting in solitude, on the other hand, is 'self-time', which leads to improvements in one's life, helps solve problems, and brings long-term happiness to the entire family. Both have their place in life.

Introspection is a powerful technique that leads to increased awareness about oneself and one's strengths and limitations. Self-analysis leads to better responses and adjustment to various situations, thus leading to improvement in the quality of one's life.

Introspection is more fruitful when attempted at a fixed place (preferably secluded) daily for at least a few minutes, sans the intrusion of gadgets. It helps to note down one's observations and thoughts. Initially, this exercise in soul-searching may be boring, but it soon becomes a routine that one longs for.

A person caught in a relentless cycle of busyness that has no place for me-time, or more importantly self-time, eventually experiences a condition of emotional and physical exhaustion called 'burnout'. The individual remains frustrated and irritable, or demonstrates zombie-like behaviour such as emotionally blunted responses, lack of motivation and detachment from immediate surroundings. There is a loss of interest in the gadgets that one couldn't do without earlier, and there is no pleasure to be found in work, affecting efficiency. The person experiences a sense of worthlessness and symptoms of either or both anxiety and depression, sometimes leading to suicidal tendencies. Regular balancing acts of introspection and revitalization ensure that such a situation does not arise.

Being too busy is injurious to our bodies and our relationships. Chronic stress is majorly detrimental to our health; it can cause long-term brain damage. Physical manifestations are the first sign—muscular pain and spasms, restlessness, headaches, fatigue, altered libido and bowel movements, and hypertension.

Its impact on emotional health is no less. The signs include indecisiveness, distress, anxiety, feelings of inadequacy and incompetence, anger, frustration, hopelessness, loneliness, and the guilt of not fulfilling one's role or maintaining relationships. The person is dogged by the fear of being judged as worthless by society.

Essentially, being busy leads to a lack of time and energy—the most important ingredients needed to sustain relationships. One may be physically present but emotionally and mentally distant, with all of one's thoughts revolving around work. Generally, family members and close friends are flexible, but if one is chronically busy, they start feeling ignored and redundant. This can lead to regular altercations and distancing. Relationships go haywire; the willingness to compromise and forgive eventually vanishes.

Sometimes, busyness becomes an excuse to avoid actual problems, like a bad relationship. But it's like burying the head in sand—the problem not only persists but slowly takes a monstruous shape, requiring more time and energy to be sorted out.

Eventually, one's profession, which is the primary reason for busyness, also suffers. A person experiencing burnout can hardly generate new ideas; besides, exhaustion increases injury hazards too. Ultimately, society is deprived of the energies of relevant individuals.

The Way Out

It is true that we live in a time that is dominated by the idea of speed. It is equally true that existing and living are very different concepts. Being excessively busy is usually the outcome of our desire to feel worthy, valuable and connected, but it can leave us feeling isolated, exhausted and inadequate; so much so that slowing down feels unnatural.

The first obstacle in breaking the shackles of busyness is overcoming the guilt associated with being free to do things other than work, especially for women. They often feel compelled to overwork due to social conditioning. Leaving certain tasks unfinished induces a much stronger sense of guilt in women in comparison to men. An awareness of the positive impacts that reducing one's workload has on work, relationships and the family's happiness should help in overcoming this barrier.

There is always strong resistance when the status quo is altered, be it from the self, dependent family members or colleagues. An assurance about your availability if a situation arises may help deal with the initial resistance. With time, everyone gets accustomed to the new reality that your happiness lies in being less busy.

The quest for perfection and micromanagement is a hindrance to freedom. There is greater happiness and productivity all around when the controlling instinct is curbed. Delegate responsibilities, ask for help from family members, or engage help (especially new mothers). Downsize housekeeping expectations. Similarly, avoid overparenting and trying to make your child an all-rounder.

To restore work–life balance, it is necessary to comprehend how your time is being spent and to reorganize your priorities. Learn to recognize the trivial and be assertive in saying no to time-consuming activities that are not in your sphere of interest. Avoid people who eat into your time like parasites.

Carve out self-time in small chunks and gradually increase it. It takes time to adjust to a new routine as older ways are deeply embedded in the subconscious. It takes self-compassion, practice and patience to break human inertia. Make to-do lists to think about what you *need* to do versus what you'd *like* to do. Self-time is a need, not an option.

Disconnecting from the distracting screen or gadgets during family and recreation time is a vital step—cultivate the idea of a 'device-free dinner' as the family's bonding time.

There's a difference between use and abuse of gadgets. The former comprises time-saving options like Internet banking, automated bill payments and online shopping. On the other hand, the fear of missing out, or FOMO, a phenomenon generated by the insatiable social media, exemplifies the abuse of gadgets. Try disconnecting for a while and you will see the reality of the world. Both your health and happiness quotient will increase. Life will once again gain a human touch.

Similarly, reducing travelling time between home and work would be beneficial to you and the family. In this era of constant job changes, this comfort may be difficult to achieve but worth exploring. For instance, if financially feasible, one of the spouses can explore this option, thus helping both the self and the family.

Once the time saved is used to connect with the self and with the family, and a pattern of work, recreation (outings, hobbies) and introspection is created, the rejuvenation experienced will overcome any resistance to change. Life will begin anew on an even more promising note.

4

Bound Together, Forever

In the past three decades, Indian society has undergone many changes, but one aspect that remains largely unchanged is its preoccupation with marriage. For most people, marriage continues to be the building block and bulwark of society. Some see it as a means of perpetuating their lineage, others a way of avoiding loneliness by finding the sort of companionship that can provide emotional and social security, and physical and psychological well-being.

What has changed in our times is the younger generation's clear-cut expectations from marriage and the partner they seek—whether through 'arranged marriage' or 'love marriage', as the terms go.

This significant life event affects not just the couple but also their respective families, friends and associates; they all need to get used to the new reality, which is not always a smooth affair. But, as has been said, change is the only constant in life.

Not all marriages are happy, and unhappy marriages become major stressors, particularly for women, who find themselves having to make more adjustments. In fact, both the 'journey towards marriage' and post-marriage life can get stressful, not only for the individuals concerned but for their near and dear ones, too. In fact, getting married is considered one of the most stressful events in life.

Journey towards Marriage

As soon as the family utters the m-word—marriage—stress can set in. For youngsters who spend longer periods pursuing higher education to land their dream job, the prospect of marriage at a conventionally 'proper' age acts as a stressor. Many of them view marriage as a speed-breaker or an end point that will force them to abandon their goals, get 'settled' and play it safe.

For young women from middle-class families in urban India who experience freedom in their parental homes, marriage can spell uncertainty—will they be able to retain their ambitions, their very personality; will they get a life partner who sees them for who they are? They see enough examples of marriages gone sour on this account, which adds to the already existing dilemma and stress.

But there is no one script for marriage—it is what we make of it. It starts from a position of respect for each other. Just as travel across different terrains requires different sets of driving skills, marital relationship, too, requires constant fine-tuning and commitment, ignoring petty issues and accommodating other viewpoints. Learning from others' mistakes helps.

The search for a perfect bride or groom through the system of arranged marriage is often overshadowed by the family's calculations regarding looks and dowry, with women often facing the trauma of rejection. Sometimes, young men and women who may be pursuing their hearts' desire elsewhere are forced into arranged marriages by their families. Moreover, the courtship period, often permitted only in a controlled environment, doesn't give the couple much insight into each other's personalities. All these situations create pressure.

The perceived gap between a dream match and the real prospect, and worries about previous love affair(s) casting a shadow on one's married life are other important stressors. The number of rejections faced is also a significant stressor, especially for those who have body image issues, whether they are men or women.

'Love relationships', too, may lead to tremendous strain. Often, couples find themselves in the difficult position of having to choose between parents and the companion. Making the decision is not easy—having a discussion with close and supportive people who may help one see the larger picture may not be a bad idea.

In the conventional view of marriage, all roles and functions are prescriptive, leaving little room for self-expression. In some cases, youngsters who have led a cocooned existence and have soft-focus ideas of the perfect romance in marriage are totally unprepared for the real thing. In all these cases, they may lack an awareness of what is essential for a strong relationship. They may be unable to see the beauty of negotiating situations based on affection, concern and respect for each other.

In a time of flux, when rigid gender roles are gradually giving way, it is important for people across generations to internalize several lessons, one of them being that women cannot always be expected to bear the brunt of sacrifice. Another is that a strong man is one who supports his wife's professional aspirations and is not intimidated by them.

Besides, household tasks are also gradually becoming a 'unisex' preserve in the urban universe. All these aspects play out in present-day marriages.

Marital Life

Marriage has a positive or negative influence on many spheres of life, depending on the temperament and expectations of the spouses and significant family members.

The gap between expectations and preconceived notions and realities of daily routines, childrearing, finances, food habits and recreational choices can become sore spots in a marital relationship. Conflicts can be decreased or avoided if the spouses and the family members know that they need to regularly fine-tune themselves. It takes equal effort from both to maintain equilibrium—for instance, both need to make the transition from singlehood to marriage by calibrating the time spent with friends and getting used to a universe of new relationships.

For some, caring and adjusting comes naturally, but for others, it requires effort. Sacrifice is not and should not be treated as a sign of weakness; rather, it's a respectable quality. Adjustment requires changing oneself. It requires give and take, which may not be apportioned equally at all times, but it should not just be one spouse who is always contributing more. The couple should not get caught up in issues such as who should make the first move, and how soon and to what extent it should be made. For either one to 'just do it' requires understanding between the two.

The In-Laws

In our society, you don't just get married to an individual; you get married to their families as well. In joint families, adults may have a more conventional worldview, so some supple navigation is required on the part of a young couple to ensure that no one feels slighted. Creating healthy boundaries in relationships with both sets of in-laws can be challenging as everyone's wishes and ideas need attention.

Couples would do well to jointly decide what to ignore or heed and to what extent, without personalizing the situation, and to learn the art of treating in-laws on both sides with equal concern. Elders, too, should realize that it is not the responsibility of the young to adjust all the time.

Behavioural Changes

Presenting one's best side for a couple of hours during courtship is easy; keeping it up 24/7 is impossible. Habits that irritate others will eventually be noticed more frequently. However, curb your instinct to change your partner's behaviour immediately. Partners who feel loved will wish to change on their own over time. Making such issues personal is always counterproductive, especially if they concern aspects with strong emotional content, like religion and customs.

Lack of positive communication between a couple is as common a stressor as a surfeit of negative communication. Listening attentively, sharing information and decision-making responsibilities, and being encouraging, appreciative and physically demonstrative help cement a relationship. Constantly questioning, arguing, criticizing and being secretive eats away at the relationship and may even lead to mental health issues.

Work-Life Balance

Demanding jobs that drain time and energy are a reality of our times. This may lead to neglect on the home front. In the case of a working couple, and also when one of the spouses is not working, the task of shouldering responsibilities becomes skewed. The problem is compounded if the spouses are in different cities. Existing issues get exacerbated, and the connection that is so essential for a healthy relationship weakens. Professional performance suffers as well. This causes all-round stress.

Acknowledging the need, and showing willingness, to connect with each other is the first step in nurturing and maintaining a relationship, be it regular communication about handling responsibilities, concern for each other's professional issues, taking time out for each other, or coming up with surprise outings and breaks, often with the family. It is equally important for the couple to realize the value of self-time, which rejuvenates the individual as well as the relationship. This includes self-awareness of excessive screen time, which eats into the relationship, and the maturity to use gadgets in ways that promote closeness. All this is part of a contemporary couple's commitment to their marital universe.

Incompatibilities

Issues stemming from temperament, lifestyle choices, and sexual and financial outlook can test a marriage. For instance, how do an introvert and an extrovert find common ground? When a workaholic marries a person who believes in a strict nine-to-five routine, how do they iron out early pinpricks? Women who have experienced the same upbringing as men in their parental home—how do they perceive the marital relationship, and how are they perceived? How do a spendthrift and a compulsive saver build their relationship?

The wider the gap, the more fixed the traits and higher the chances of pressure. Repeated comments to change one's personality make the problem worse. Initially, giving one's spouse space to express themselves is sensible, and an acceptance of differing lifestyle choices shows big-heartedness.

What the couple can do is identify crucial aspects on which it would be better for both to be on the same wavelength, such as financial planning. They should ideally agree upon securing the family's core financial strength (and planning budgets), and beyond that, accept the freedom of the other to express their lifestyle. Enjoying the fruits of the money earned also brings happiness.

Being opinionated can be problematic; there has to be a readiness to meet the other person halfway. However, if problems persist, then intervention by well-wishers or professionals may be required. Sexual incompatibility or denying sexual intimacy is a major stressor among couples. A good sexual life is an important ingredient of bonding; the lack of it gives rise to a feeling of being unloved and unappreciated, and a desire to find that satisfaction elsewhere. Sexual frustration can lead to emotional and, eventually, physical separation. Attempting to meet each other halfway can help, and so can discussing issues such as decreased libido (due to age, responsibilities, etc.) unhesitatingly. Or, if the couple so feels, they can seek professional help for marital or sexual counselling.

Parenting

Deciding whether and when to have children can be difficult when the spouses are not of the same view. Problems in conceiving, miscarriages, having children with disability, or the loss of a child—these are traumatic experiences that often lead to recriminations. Differing parenting styles, too, are a constant source of altercations.

Life alters once children arrive. Responsibilities increase, and couples fall back on a traditional division of labour that impacts women more, whether they are homemakers or professionals. Being supportive in handling duties can propel the relationship in a positive direction.

Disparity in childrearing approaches is a constant source of disagreement. Lack of time for children is an added pressure. Fighting in front of children is a strict no-no, for it affects their psyche. Parents should remember that their egoistic views can have a problematic effect on their children.

The Pressure of Poor Health and Difficult Times

Poor professional, physical or emotional health puts added pressure on marriage, affecting togetherness. Women generally are more communicative, while men try to deal with the pressure on their own (self-medicating or taking to alcohol and smoking). Differences in approaching the issue may create discord.

The question is, is companionship meant only for happy times? Empathy is an important ingredient in a healthy relationship, and the assurance of getting through a crisis as a family helps the relationship in the long run.

During difficult times, communication and support are essential. They help one to both identify problem areas and to try to change one's life patterns. For instance, listing bothersome issues and seeking to reach middle ground is one way (such as, between total abstinence and daily imbibing, coming to the decision to limit drinking to once a week), as is recognizing that some issues are non-negotiable (such as treating the partner's parents with contempt). Knowing when to seek professional aid is also important.

Playing the blame game, on the other hand, can create a spiral of negativity and lead to an immensely stressful cycle of irreconcilable differences, which could end up in separation and divorce.

The bottom line is, keeping a marriage alive is possible if both the spouses wish it and are ready to jointly face the challenges that come their way.

5

The Side Effects of Temptation

Whenever and wherever the subject of extramarital affairs comes up, it is usually accompanied by the following words—cheating, unfaithfulness, infidelity, betrayal, deceitfulness, disloyalty, dishonesty, treachery and illicit relationships. These terms demonstrate the negativity that is associated with extramarital affairs. Anything that weakens the institution of marriage is viewed suspiciously by large sections of society.

There is a view that extramarital affairs are on the rise in urban India and that several factors are responsible for it, such as the seductive influence of present-day media and celebrity lifestyles, the growing emphasis on individual desires, personal communication being made easy by technology, and increased proximity between the sexes. However, beyond all these aspects is the human factor—human intent—which is at the core of all things.

The Question Is, Why?

On any given day, the media is full of titillating stories about the extramarital affairs of celebs, ranging from politicians and famous business persons to sportspersons and actors. Often, a friends' get-together becomes a gossip session about who in their circle is having an affair. Eyebrows are raised if it is someone who seems to have a perfect marriage.

Wrong. It just *seems* perfect. Something is wrong in that marriage; there is definitely some kind of psychological struggle underway. In my practice, I have observed that usually there can be one or more of these factors at play— early marriage, incompatibility, decreased sexual intimacy (due to a mismatch in libido or preoccupation with work), monotony and boredom in the relationship, a longing for excitement and to 'feel alive', even peer pressure sometimes. Mostly, extramarital relationships are a result of chronic marital maladjustment coupled with a midlife crisis and easy opportunity.

As a society, we are at a juncture where greater urbanization and mobility, loosening of traditional mores, changing gender equations, a rising sense of individualism and aspirations, combined with increasing means of communication, have impacted just about every aspect of our lives, including the traditional idea of marriage.

A marriage lacking consent on one or both sides and marked by emotional disconnect; personality issues like poor adjustment capabilities, and verbally and physically abusive behaviour; and different priorities and interests—all these are factors that could lead to marital discord. When one partner goes to court to seek a separation, a vacuum is created. In such a troubled state, the tendency is to share one's feelings, and if the confidante is of the opposite sex, same age group and is accessible and empathetic on account of personal emotional traumas, the chances of a friendship growing into an extramarital relationship increase.

In marriages that may be drifting after a positive beginning, discontent followed by indifference may create a situation where the marriage does not seem worth it. It is at that point precisely that the couple needs to communicate with each other, and remember the trust they had placed in each other years ago. This communication is generally facilitated by children, friends or professionals. Trust and respect, once lost, are hard to regain.

Therefore, it's important to introspect on what one wants—a distraction that initially makes one feel good or to rekindle the connection that had once been part of the marriage. That can only happen when companionship and intimacy become a priority for the couple once again, no matter what the hassles of daily living are.

The couple needs to take some steps consciously—change troubling habits, do things together, make every effort to rekindle their sex life and sense of humour. All these elements contribute to the longevity of a relationship. Most of all, the knowledge that the bond between them is still strong will keep the marriage alive.

A healthy companionship is one in which partners are willing to make adjustments and readjustments as the situation requires—not just one person all the time, but both. The tendency to bury unresolved issues, which is passivity, does not work. As the discomfort increases, the passivity eventually turns into aggressiveness, towards the self or others. The best option is to be assertive and bring out issues into the open. Once things cool down, the couple can discuss the issues with an intent to begin anew.

The effort should be to have a relationship in which communication lines with the partner are always open, allowing the freedom to express thoughts, concerns and emotions. Expressing oneself candidly in a non-harmful way draws new boundaries. At such a juncture where solutions are not easy to find, couples can always turn to trusted family members, friends or a professional to help them through that learning curve.

The best of marriages falter at times because the learning curve of one partner outstrips the other. Only when both partners feel a sense of purpose and joy in their personal quests will they be secure and companionable. That personal quest can be anything that interests them—studying, teaching, cooking, baking, designing, volunteering for a cause or joining a group activity, to name a few.

With growing responsibilities, such as parenthood and the demands of the job, physical intimacy may lessen, leading to a general cooling off. Whatever the circumstances, a feeling of being ignored should not be created. Someone who feels that their partner is too wrapped up in other things to sense the aloofness creeping in should convey it in so many words. Communication, to get back into the act and to find a middle ground, is all-important.

In many cases, the timing of sexual desire may not match, which is also a cause for frustration as physical intimacy is an important element of a happy marriage. How open the couple is to discussing their sexual needs and frustrations and how willing they are to reach a solution are important.

If a partner realizes that the other is making an effort to change and provide sexual satisfaction, and if intimacy is accompanied by emotional conversations, it strengthens the connection between partners. The warmth of touch is essential—hugs and kisses reaffirm closeness.

On the other hand, if a couple is not open to discussing these issues, and if annoyance starts building up in one partner, who gets swayed on hearing friends talk about their affairs, a new train of thought could be started.

Here it would be wise to pause and ask yourself a few questions—what is the cost of the extramarital affair in terms of the impact on self and family that the friend is paying? Is the impulse to snatch momentary pleasure worth putting the marriage at risk, especially if there are aspects in which there is still a connection?

The times we live in emphasize speed. 'Live in the moment, live for yourself' is the theme. More and more men and women are working together in professional environments and socializing, which may be a new and exhilarating experience for them. Impulsiveness is the name of the game, as is the idea of being 'modern' about casual relationships. The air of permissiveness and urban anonymity, ever-increasing dating apps and sites coupled with the lure of a smartphone seemingly allow one to explore a private world of fantasies for a while, without impacting the primary relationship.

Is it true, though, that the primary relationship will stay unaffected?

The next question is—how well do you know yourself?

In my practice, I have come across cases where extramarital affairs were started purely for the sexual aspect; in others, the motivation was to take revenge on the spouse. Some people saw office flings as a way to get ahead professionally. Others had the desire to be seen and appreciated again because they felt invisible in their marital relationship.

Many times, people start an extramarital affair thinking it's a casual fling. They are not aware that any relationship can develop intensely emotional undertones that can precipitate extreme acts. It may be casual for one but not for the other person—daily news reports about crimes of passion are testament to this reality. Sometimes, these affairs are also a way of duping people at their most vulnerable. Some people even end up taking their lives, not knowing how to set things right. The point is that there is never anything casual about a so-called casual extramarital relationship. Every relationship extracts a price.

What is passable in some marriages is anathema to others. In some marriages, a partner flirting with the opposite sex may not offend the spouse; in some, it's a no-no. Responses vary depending on temperament, age, duration of the marriage, socio-economic background and cultural milieu.

What is normal is not the issue; what is dangerous and harmful to a particular relationship is the question. Sometimes it's healthier to state openly if one finds another person attractive while acknowledging one's boundaries. For, along with love and respect, a marriage is about commitment.

After the Affair

The consequences of an extramarital affair are many—the person who has stepped out of marital bounds is weighed down by it eventually. Denial, grief, remorse and aggression are natural outcomes. The spouse and the family, particularly children, are affected. Even friends find themselves divided in support of one or the other.

The irony is that the affair that was started to make one feel good and lighter becomes intensely stressful. There is the fear of being discovered, of accidentally becoming pregnant, of someone else reading messages, and of being blackmailed with images of intimacy captured on the ubiquitous smartphone, for instance. In case of the latter, it is better to come clean with the spouse and report the matter to the police to protect oneself from or end the blackmail.

On discovery, which is inevitable, if the couple still wants to work it out, the frayed relationship needs to be mended. It is easier said than done.

Initially, anger is at its peak and the chances of patching up seem remote. However, with time, depending on the intent to mend fences, the wounds may start healing, though it requires enormous patience and effort to reestablish trust. For instance, if the person was having an affair with a colleague, moving out of that office would demonstrate an intent to work on the marital relationship. Discussing and modifying the correctable reasons behind drifting apart would help in decreasing the conflict. Guidance from empathetic family members and counselling may help in tiding over the crisis. Guilt resolution and rebuilding trust takes a while, as does resolving the grief associated with a break-up.

Sometimes, a couple may find it hard to get past the crisis. Once the rift becomes irrevocable, there's no point continuing to live under one roof acrimoniously. It is better to go your separate ways. This conversation is not easy to initiate, and the partners must ensure that children are not used as a tool of revenge, for it can scar them for a lifetime.

The worrying aspect is the impact of one partner's extramarital affair on the other. It can be a roller coaster of emotions, with the faithful partner going from starting arguments to withdrawal and depression, resorting to drugs, or developing suicidal or homicidal thoughts. Some may blame themselves for the partner's affair, feel a lack of self-esteem, or even be guilt-ridden enough to think extreme thoughts.

Apart from compulsive sexual behaviour or an excitement-driven personality, any extramarital affair denotes an underlying problem in marital relations to which both partners have contributed, intentionally or unintentionally. Introspection is key to moving on. Although it is not easy, one's ego has to be kept aside. Humans possess excellent cognitive abilities and have the capacity to change themselves.

Uncovering the reasons and course correction take time and energy; both require patience and trust. Particularly after a crisis like this, it is important for a couple to clear the air by talking things out—what they mean to each other, where they slipped and the insecurities that one expects the other to understand, especially those like being taken for granted.

If the discussion becomes a medium of humiliation, then the whole purpose of the talk is lost. If the couple is able to comprehend that marriage is at all times work in progress, there is hope for them. Making oneself attractive to the partner once again is part of it, as is the resolve to be a witness to the other's life again.

6

The Motherhood Experience

'So, when are you giving us the good news?' This is the one question that newly-wed couples can be asked anywhere, anytime in India.

Over several decades, as smaller, nuclear families have become the norm among the middle class, especially in urban India, couples have largely started choosing what they think is the right time for them to start a family.

Like most life events that are simultaneously exciting and stressful for the changes and adjustments they herald, the decision to get pregnant can be just as stressful as the pregnancy itself. The term 'pregnancy anxiety' encompasses all kinds of worries—about one's own and the baby's health, hospital and healthcare experiences, imminent childbirth and parenting.

The fact that during pregnancy, a majority of women experience low to moderate stress, and a small percentage experience high levels of stress, is well researched.[10] It occurs

---

[10] Dunkel Schetter, Christine, and Lynlee R. Tanner, 'Anxiety, Depression and Stress in Pregnancy: Implications for Mothers, Children, Research, and Practice', *Current Opinion in Psychiatry*, Vol. 25, No. 2, 2012,

due to a complex interplay of factors, such as pre-pregnancy predisposition to anxiety and depression, and social, familial, financial and environmental conditions during pregnancy.

Preparing for Pregnancy

The present-day generation in urban India has its own way of easing into new roles. Couples believe that it is important for them to get used to the role of a spouse and develop a strong understanding and companionship before becoming parents. The thought behind this is that a new life should be brought into the world only when both partners are satisfied about the enduring nature of their relationship. Other people may warn about the biological clock ticking away and the problems and complications that accompany late pregnancy. They may point out that life is not linear; so many things happen simultaneously and have to be dealt with. But when to have the child is something that the couple needs to decide jointly.

Moreover, the couple feels the need to be financially steady, which may be tied to certain milestones such as reaching a certain professional level, owning a house, having enough resources for the child's education, and possessing

---

pp. 141–8, https://tinyurl.com/326mxaen. Accessed on 12 March 2024; Woods, Sarah M., et al., 'Psychosocial Stress During Pregnancy', *American Journal of Obstetrics and Gynecology*, Vol. 202, No. 1, 2010, pp. 61.e1–7, https://tinyurl.com/2bb8yn52. Accessed on 12 March 2024; Bleker, Laura S., Susanne R. de Rooij and Tessa J. Roseboom, 'Prenatal Psychological Stress Exposure and Neurodevelopment and Health of Children', *International Journal of Environmental Research and Public Health*, Vol. 16, No. 19, 2019, p. 3657, https://tinyurl.com/bdhesnd7. Accessed on 12 March 2024.

other material comforts. Considering that the milestones shift every now and then, seeking that 'perfect time' can generate its own anxiety.

For many, the desire to be parents is a natural progression from marriage, but the decision to get pregnant can still be stressful. Couples need to be mentally prepared for the changes and responsibilities associated with pregnancy and childrearing.

Other times, the anxiety stems from the fact that the partners don't share the same view about having children. Every apprehension needs to be discussed with an open mind: whether to be a parent or not; if not, why not; if yes, what the right time is; how difficult it is to bring up a child; what the problems faced are; and, most importantly, what the positives of being a parent are and what difference a child can make to one's life. Once the decision is made, the couple should face every new situation with the conviction that it's worth it.

Common Worries during Pregnancy

The hormonal changes during pregnancy, when coupled with the person's situation, unleash a cocktail of emotions—one is now happy, now calm, now in a blue mood, now stressed—depending on several factors. It could be the mother's first pregnancy, hence the anxiety of the unknown; it could be an unplanned, unwanted pregnancy or a much longed-for pregnancy after previous negative experiences. For some, there's the added pressure of bearing a male child, if the couple or the relatives have a conservative mindset. And, in today's times, the financial pressure is never too far.

For some, the stress begins when they find out that they

are pregnant. Anxieties crowd in—will they reach full term safely, have an easy delivery, be good parents? Then there are the worries about one's career, the changes in physical appearance, less time for the self and family, which give rise to a feeling of being constantly rushed off one's feet.

At such times, books on pregnancy and the Internet may be helpful, but the support and understanding of experienced people close to the couple is invaluable—they can convey to the expectant parents that what they are going through is a universal life event.

If it is the first pregnancy, the couple's focus is on what to do and what not to do—what type of food to eat, what activities to pursue or avoid, how to protect the mother from disease so that the child faces no problems, etc.

There is a surfeit of information at hand, particularly online, but it would be wise to share your daily experiences with a close friend or relative who has experienced motherhood. For sound medical advice, there is always the doctor.

Dealing with the discomforts associated with different stages of pregnancy, like morning sickness, constipation, frequent urination, backache, tiredness and mood swings, is not easy, especially if it's the first or a difficult pregnancy. Daily and recreational activities get restricted. Weight gain leads to breathing and sleeping difficulties, and that can be troublesome. But it is helpful to remember that these physiological changes are short-lived and mostly reversible.

Limitation of sexual activity during the first trimester and advanced pregnancy due to reasons including doctor's advice, fear of harming the child, and so on can be frustrating. But it's only a matter of time. Physical contact in the form of kissing and hugging provides much warmth. Self-stimulatory activity (masturbation) is an alternative.

Visits to the doctor's clinic and labs and the expenditure they entail can also cause stress. The good thing is that the frequency of visits is not high, unless it's a complicated pregnancy. Choosing a doctor nearby is sensible, and appointments can be combined with other activities like a chore or recreational activity. These days, home collection services are available for most blood tests, making the entire process less stressful.

It is a well-established fact that the foetus is impacted by the mother's frame of mind. Hence, pregnant women are advised to be in a positive frame of mind at such times. In the face of negative events—job loss, indifferent behaviour of the partner, death in the family or even a pandemic, as was witnessed recently—the rule of thumb is to manage the issues that can be dealt with. For instance, if the couple stays in a neighbourhood that lacks several amenities, the expectant mother can spend some time at her maternal home. As for circumstances beyond their control, a couple should try to mentally distance themselves from them.

The timing and magnitude of stress impacts the outcome of pregnancy. Stress can cause pregnancy hypertension and diabetes, and it can weaken the mother's immune system. It can also lead to miscarriage or preterm birth of a baby with low birth weight, which has far-reaching consequences like delayed development milestones and cognitive, emotional and behavioural disorders. That is how a vicious cycle of stress is created.

To be in a positive and relaxed frame of mind is the best counter to stress. Connecting with relatives and friends who have a positive mindset, spending time with people who are on the same wavelength and with whom you can laugh, listening to soothing music, reading books that have a calming effect, playing board games and the like help with that.

Permitted yoga and physical exercises that do not increase abdominal pressure are also helpful. Regular walks are beneficial. The temptation to 'relax' with a cigarette or alcohol should be firmly avoided. Appropriate and timely professional help, prescribed medications, counselling and social support are helpful in fighting back stress in extreme cases.

The partner's steadfast support is essential. It is important that he considers himself equally invested in the journey to parenthood. Besides, pregnancy is not an illness and should not be treated like one. That will reduce worries.

Job versus Parenthood

It is a striking irony that society expects a woman to fulfil the role of a mother prescribed for her culturally, but in the contemporary workspace, that very social obligation is considered as a black mark on a woman's career, signalling her lack of commitment to work as opposed to the ambition of a male colleague. Many young women professionals also see it as such. Although maternity leave is mandatory, many companies try to circumvent it with some excuse or the other, seeing it as a drain on them. All this creates much stress for the expectant mother and for the family, as many households are dependent on a dual source of income.

These situations demand innovative solutions. An arrangement with the employer whereby working from home some days a week becomes an option post delivery, and arrangements at home whereby one's partner, parents, relatives and domestic staff take on some chores are worth exploring. With a workable plan in place, the expectant mother will be less worried.

Couples starting families may have some self-doubt—will they be good parents? They are aware that they will be required to take on multiple roles, which were earlier distributed across a joint family. They need to understand that there's a difference between good and perfect parenting—good parenting is easy, while perfect parenting is an unachievable, stressful goal. Focussing on precise efforts for a perfect result cannot hold a candle to raising a child with love, warmth and care. A large part of good parenting is determined by common sense, and elders and friends are always around to help with timely tips. These days, there are also many digital parental support groups that parents can join to share their experiences and learn from others.

Changes in the Life of Expectant Parents

Pregnancy changes the lives of both partners. While it is the wife who physiologically experiences pregnancy, the husband goes through it emotionally and mentally. A caring husband knows he has to be his wife's biggest support through her ups and downs. During this time, he can mentally prepare himself for parenthood, not just out of duty but because he wants to. His supportive role is important in determining the family's stress level as a whole.

Pregnancy alters the partner's life as well—he may not be able to devote extra time to his profession or to himself, but he can learn to adjust his schedule so that his priorities can be accomplished.

That said, he too needs some social support during this time. If he is unable to meet friends regularly, he can connect with them digitally. Since he will be spending more time at home, he can start engaging in his preferred activities, like exercising or other hobbies, accordingly.

If it is the second pregnancy, the couple should ensure that the older child does not feel excluded from the preparations for the new child, and is made to feel like an integral part of the journey. The elders will need to be big-hearted to understand the situation and adjust accordingly.

Reducing Stress

Here is a list of things a couple can do to deal with stress during pregnancy:

- Identify (perhaps in writing) your stress triggers and try to overcome or sidestep them.
- Slow down, go easy on the desire to chase perfection at work.
- If tired, don't feel responsible for every household chore. Leave some for the future.
- Pamper yourself whenever possible.
- Take adequate rest and sleep.
- Do yoga, meditation or some exercise (to the extent permitted) to reduce pregnancy stress and common pregnancy discomforts. Take professional help if in doubt.
- Engage in your favourite activities—reading, listening to music, watching TV or pursuing a hobby.
- Enrol for childbirth and post-delivery education classes.

- Try not to spend too much time online to get information, much of which is unauthenticated. Experienced people and medical professionals around you can offer better advice.

If a predisposition to stress is identified pre-pregnancy, efforts should be made to strengthen the psychosocial resources of the expectant mother at the earliest opportunity. If the symptoms escalate to indicate depression or anxiety, professional help—counselling and safe medication—may become essential.

Stress during pregnancy has both short-term and long-term impacts on the mother, the baby and eventually the whole family, so it is imperative to manage it properly at all stages. That is when pregnancy becomes a worthwhile journey of discovery.

7

Pressure of Procreation

'Why haven't you given us any good news? Is it that you don't want to have or that you can't have children?' This is a question that couples, and especially women, routinely face in India.

Traditionally, getting married and having children are taken for granted. To many, biological children signify the perpetuation of their lineage and are considered crucial support for ageing parents. The idea that a married couple may choose not to have children is still unfamiliar to considerable sections of Indian society, to whom a childless marriage is not a 'fruitful' marriage. Often, the inability to conceive is stigmatized.

Many couples are unable to have children, for they suffer from infertility. Scientifically, infertility is defined as the inability to conceive despite having frequent, carefully timed, unprotected intercourse for at least a year. Since it is women who get pregnant, traditionally they have had to bear the brunt of societal prejudice, even though the cause of infertility may lie in either or both partners.

A couple that has failed to conceive even once suffers from primary infertility, which is cause for stress, especially if the partners greatly desire to have their own biological children. Failure to conceive again is a case of secondary infertility, which puts pressure on a couple that may have suffered an earlier miscarriage or a sudden death of a child, or desires a sibling for their child with disability. In a traditional set-up, a couple with one daughter comes under pressure to try for a male child.

The fertility rate in India (number of children born per woman) has been on the decline, falling from 4.97 during 1975–80 to 2.3 in 2015–20, and is projected to come down to 2.1 by 2025–30, and 1.86 by 2045–50.[11] This is the usual progression associated with urbanizing societies.

In urban India, infertility affects one out of six couples,[12] and has significant social, psychological, interpersonal and financial consequences. Earlier, it was considered a matter of shame, but now, more and more couples are willing to discuss their problems openly. This is a positive development.

Causes of Infertility

There can be physiological and anatomical impediments to conception. In the case of females, all the steps during ovulation and fertilization need to occur correctly. As for males, the semen should have enough motile sperms for fertility. Investigations, including blood tests, semen

---

[11]Population Division, Department of Social and Economic Affairs, United Nations, *World Population Prospects: The 2017 Revision*, 2017, https://tinyurl.com/5e9er9sh. Accessed on 12 March 2024.

[12]Shiraz, Zarafshan, 'Most Common Causes of Low Sperm Count in Men and Female Infertility in India', *Hindustan Times*, 30 January 2023, https://tinyurl.com/mry8feak. Accessed on 12 March 2024.

analysis, and imaging (ultrasound, X-ray, etc.), are required to detect the exact cause of failure to conceive.

Beyond this, research has revealed an association between primary infertility and factors such as living in nuclear families, increasing employment of women, high levels of education, socio-economic status, obesity, stress and depression.[13]

A mix of lifestyle and environmental factors impact fertility.[14] These include:

- a delayed marriage;
- postponing parenthood;
- excessively high or low weight;
- alcohol consumption and smoking;
- stress and anxiety;
- vehicular pollution;
- food grown with pesticides;
- some illnesses, medications and treatment modalities (as in the case of cancer);
- sexually transmitted diseases owing to unprotected sex or overuse of emergency contraceptives;
- low sexual frequency;

---

[13] Katole, Ashwini, and Ajeet Saoji, 'Prevalence of Primary Infertility and Its Associated Risk Factors in Urban Population of Central India: A Community-Based Cross-Sectional Study', *Indian Journal of Community Medicine*, Vol. 44, No. 4, 2019, pp. 337–41, https://tinyurl.com/5dr28fmy. Accessed on 12 March 2024.

[14] Bala, Renu, et al., 'Environment, Lifestyle, and Female Infertility', *Reproductive Sciences*, Vol. 28, 2021, pp. 617–38, https://tinyurl.com/2uauhkzp. Accessed on 12 March 2024; Sharpe, Richard M., 'Lifestyle and Environmental Contribution to Male Infertility', *British Medical Bulletin*, Vol. 56, No. 3, 2000, pp. 630–42, https://tinyurl.com/5xf7fuuc. Accessed on 12 March 2024.

- overexposure to heat (saunas or tight undergarments) in the case of men; and
- regular strenuous exercise by women.

The realization that lifestyle affects the ability to conceive often makes a couple feel guilty. But brooding may further hamper the efforts to conceive and cause more stress. It is better to look ahead and take corrective action, such as:

- regular intercourse, especially around ovulation time;
- leading a healthy and balanced life;
- stopping fertility-impacting medications (bodybuilding products, prolonged use of steroids, hormonal pills) and replacing these with alternatives after consulting one's doctor; and
- remaining stress-free as far as possible by adopting relaxation techniques, seeking counselling and/or using medication.

It is a fact that fertility tends to decline with age. It's also true that the current generation of urban Indians is increasingly veering towards late marriage and parenthood. As discussed in earlier chapters, their decisions are affected by a desire to reach a certain level of stability and confidence—emotional and financial.

Inflexible work policies, lack of childcare support in nuclear families, and the thought that it is unfair to become parents if you are not able to devote enough time to the child also play their part in the decision-making process. Moreover, as young men and women in rapidly urbanizing spaces explore several relationships, informal and formal, before finding the companionship and stability they are seeking, the decision to have children gets delayed.

In all these circumstances, they can push parenthood to a later age because of effective contraception. However, many are unaware of the impacts of advancing age on fertility. The human tendency is to think that there is enough time for everything, but one should not ignore the significance of the fact that the body has a biological mechanism, and may not function the way one wants it to by the time the professional and personal aspects are favourable.

As such, when couples pushing the age limit do decide to start a family, many face problems conceiving. Scientifically speaking, the age of 35 is termed to be advanced maternal age, and achieving motherhood after it leads to higher chances of maternal and foetal risk.[15] In many cases, such couples suffer from infertility.

Impact of Infertility

For a couple that desires children, not being able to conceive is distressing, more so for the woman who is made to feel less of a woman due to societal prejudice. If the wait for a positive result every month after repeated efforts keeps extending, the stress experienced by the couple is immense. The situation often worsens as the couple starts playing the blame game and feeling guilty over their lifestyle decisions.

In sections of urban India that are still bound by conservatism, arguments often erupt between couples even before the cause of infertility is diagnosed. At such times, the

---

[15]Committee on Clinical Consensus–Obstetrics, and Society for Maternal-Fetal Medicine, 'Pregnancy at Age 35 Years or Older', *Obstetrics & Gynecology*, Vol. 140, No. 2, 2022, https://tinyurl.com/mr2jvehk. Accessed on 12 March 2024.

patriarchal mindset rears its head even among the educated—very often the in-laws, focussed on the perpetuation of their lineage, demand that their daughters-in-law be examined, investigated and treated before their son.

In such circumstances, cases of husbands physically abusing their spouses, taking to alcohol, or having extramarital affairs are not uncommon. Women, though, often adopt a different coping mechanism: they tend to withdraw into themselves and fight shy of social contact. On the whole, childless couples suffer social deprivation and its consequences in the form of inferiority, guilt and sometimes suicidal ideas. Even if the couple's immediate families are liberal and supportive, the surrounding environment often becomes negative due to the incessant, invasive questions that are directed at them, and more so at the women: are there any relationship problems? Are there any medical problems? Who has the problem? Such questions are hurtful, and one has to learn to not react to them. Generally, they are followed by unsolicited advice from relatives, neighbours or acquaintances without consideration for the couple's troubled frame of mind.

To avoid the pressure of this constant scrutiny, couples may become secretive, excuse themselves from social scenarios, or even try to move to a different location. This deprives them of the support of the people who truly care for them.

One is not obligated to respond to everyone. Generally, the couple knows what kind of people they might encounter at a social occasion, so they can prepare themselves to handle intrusive questions. If need be, the couple should be assertive enough to say that their personal space is being intruded upon and causing them discomfort. This assertion takes considerable energy, leaving the couple drained.

What gives the couple the confidence to face any situation is each other's support. It is important to have an empathetic friend circle. Moreover, spending time with nephews, nieces or friends' children can satisfy parental urges.

Thankfully, there is a growing awareness of the fact that the problem may lie with either or both partners or none, and that, like corrective medical or surgical procedures for problems in other bodily organs, there are medications and surgeries for reproductive organs as well.

Accepting the problem is the first step to conquering it. Rather than giving in to anxiety, it is prudent to seek professional help at some point, be it for infertility or the associated mental health issues.

Even before knowing what the problem is, some couples start unproven alternative remedies, on their own or upon coercion by their families (especially the in-laws), either for fear that allopathic treatment may be too expensive or out of blind faith. It is judicious to pursue a scientific approach.

Available Treatments

The decision to pursue infertility treatment is not simple. A part of you may want to wait a bit longer in the hope of conceiving, but logic dictates that the wait has been long enough. It is perhaps wiser to not delay the treatment indefinitely, for commencing treatment at a relatively younger age means a greater chance of conception and higher quality embryo and sperm.

Before the investigations commence, the partners should assure each other that the one diagnosed with the problem will not be blamed in any way, that they are a team in this endeavour. The couple should also fully understand what the treatment entails, including the side effects.

The first step involves giving the doctor a detailed history of one's relationship and sexual activities (both past and current). Some may find this awkward and stressful. If uncomfortable, one can request an interview in the absence of the spouse. The doctors are bound by confidentiality, so one can be honest without worrying. It is important to share details truthfully as the doctor tries to build a picture of the person's life and lifestyle.

The couple can prepare a list of queries regarding the stages of treatment, related side effects, chances of success, and expenses before proceeding further. Although it's not uncommon for couples to go through periods of anxiety, regret and depression, the chances of the treatment succeeding increase when they are in a positive frame of mind.

The next question facing the couple is whether they should be investigated simultaneously or one by one. The procedures can be time-consuming and painful. Simultaneous investigation of both saves time and effort, but the question of finances is bound to come up. Often, rest is required after a procedure, and some help may be needed around the house to provide relief to the couple. Partners should be sensitive to each other during this stressful period.

Psychological turmoil, guilt, thoughts like 'I should have ordered my life differently', feelings of failure, apprehensions, helplessness and hopelessness are common emotional reactions of couples not only during treatment but also if each procedure results in failure. Mental health suffers. At times, the couple also has to deal with a lack of empathy from the persons conducting investigations and conveying results. The support of close family and friends is essential.

Depending on the cause, the treatment can be either medicinal or carried out by means of assisted reproductive technology (ART), which includes in vitro fertilization (IVF).

Assisted reproductive technology is painful for women as it involves multiple injections for stimulating ovulation. The treatment can lead to stressful complications like multiple pregnancies, bleeding and infections. Moreover, the existence of unscrupulous practices—such as uncertainty about whether the couple's own sperm and egg will be used—increases all-round stress. The clinic should be chosen with care.

While expenses increase with the complexity and multiple attempts of ART, it does not guarantee success. The uncertainty creates more stress for the couple, further decreasing the chance of conception. The stress may continue even after a positive result, in this case about the safe continuation of pregnancy.

The financial aspect of the treatment may cause the couple distress. Some sell off assets or take loans; others may resort to painful lifestyle decisions to invest in an infertility treatment whose outcome is unsure. Financial assistance from the family, if it comes, is a big gesture of support. The couple can also choose to seek treatment at government facilities, which charge less.

The cycle of uncertainty makes coping extremely difficult. It is better to jointly decide how many trials are emotionally and financially viable. This may reduce anxiety during treatments and negative outcomes. Accepting it and considering alternatives like adoption (or opting for donor sperm/egg) or even remaining childless (and working with children in several capacities) would be better for psychological health.

Beyond all this is a simple truth: if the partners care for

each other and are each other's biggest strength, there is nothing they cannot face together.

The Option of Adoption

Today, an increasing number of couples think that experiencing parenthood is more important than experiencing pregnancy, and they achieve their goal through adoption.

Among them are childless couples who do not want to experience the prolonged uncertainty of infertility treatments (the single biggest factor for adoption), single women who wish to experience motherhood, couples wanting to expand their family (for instance, those with a son wanting a daughter), adoptees who want to change the life of a child like theirs was changed years ago, and those who do so for altruistic reasons (wanting to give a child a loving environment). In some cases, the adoptee is the child of someone known, like a close family member. There are also cases where a woman goes through pregnancy for a childless family member to adopt the child. Formally recognized and legalized, this is called an open adoption, for the biological and adoptive families stay in touch.

Mostly, couples who want to adopt go through adoption agencies or child care institutions (CCIs). The child's antecedents are not revealed, hence the term 'closed adoption'. In India, CCIs are governed by the regulations of Central Adoption Resource Authority (CARA) to prevent the misuse of adoption for illegal activities. The child can be adopted from the state in which one resides, from another state or even from another country.

Adoption changes the lives of the adopted child and

adoptive parents. With the arrival of a child, the contours of a family take shape. However, in addition to the stresses commonly associated with parenthood, several emotional ups and downs linked to adoption are experienced by an adoptive parent before, during and after adoption. The child may also undergo similar turmoil. The psychological trauma is an interplay of many factors and may surface soon or long after adoption.

Before proceeding with adoption, couples and their families need to ask themselves why they want to adopt a child. Sometimes, due to the emotional upheaval caused by futile infertility treatments, a couple may decide to adopt a child without asking themselves if they have the motivation and mental preparation it requires. The decision to adopt should not be emotional; it should be well-thought-out.

The adoption procedure, too, is cumbersome and uncertain, making prospective adopters feel vulnerable at times. The denial of a request for adoption, following the evaluation of a couple's financial, medical and psychological suitability, can be devastating. Then there are the logistical aspects to consider, like legal formalities and having to travel to and stay in another city where a CCI may be based.

Familiarizing oneself with the procedure and the time it takes, in the interest of the child, is the first preparatory step. Further, the parents need to accept that they may not have access to the child's complete history, like parentage, social and medical history, and the reasons why the child was given up. Only when the parents decide that their child's origin has no bearing on how they feel about them—and accept that their child's new life begins the day they are adopted—will they be comfortable.

In the case of childless couples, the prolonged anticipation of parenthood and the excitement of adoption can give way to a feeling of sadness. This is called the post-adoption depression syndrome. The unexpected difficulties of parenthood and its responsibilities can be overwhelming. It takes the couple a while to adjust to new roles, routines and responsibilities, and they feel out of depth at times.

During this phase, many couples may question their love for the child and their parenting capabilities. They may fear discussing these issues and feel isolated, but they should realize that parenting comprises a set of skills that vary according to the child's age, and are learned through one's own experiences and those of family members and friends.

The couple faces another troubling dilemma—should the child be told about the adoption? If so, who should break the news, in what manner and when? Opinions vary on this question. Some say, why tell the child unless they come to know somehow? Others feel that the child should be told the truth at an appropriate age by the parents in a cordial atmosphere.

The best option is for parents to tell the children when they are old enough to comprehend it (any time after the child reaches the age of five). The story around the child's adoption should be kept as simple and positive as possible. Children must be given space to ask questions and express turbulent emotions. This is bound to happen at various times and at any age. Their doubts should be handled with positivity on each occasion.

Once aware of their adoption, children may feel abandoned or grieve the loss of their biological family, especially during an argumentative phase with their adoptive parents or when confronting the demands of life that seem excessive to them. The grief that they experience is very real.

Especially during adolescence, adopted children tend to mull over the circumstances surrounding their birth and adoption, often coming up with their own story full of painful emotions. Experiencing shame and loss of self-esteem, especially because society's image of their birth parents is often negative, they may secretly yearn for their birth parents and information about themselves. Often, they face identity issues, wondering if they 'fit in'. Sadness, guilt, withdrawal, aggression, self-hate and self-harm are common reactions.

There is a spectrum of difficult behaviours linked to the child's adoptive status—attachment disorders, propensity to lie, rebelling against authority, separation anxiety and major depression. There is a greater predisposition to lasting emotional trauma and a higher likelihood of behavioural, learning and attention difficulties in adopted children.[16]

The child's continuous difficulties can be stressful for the parents, who may develop a fear of rejection. Their frustrations impact the child, leading to a vicious circle of negativity. Wondering if they make good parents, at times a couple may even start questioning their decision to adopt.

They need to understand that it is not that there is a deficiency in their parenting, but that they must learn to tackle such difficult circumstances with empathy and love. For instance, adoptive parents should internalize the sensitivities of positive adoption language. This includes

---

[16]Paine, Amy L., et al., 'Charting the Trajectories of Adopted Children's Emotional and Behavioral Problems: The Impact of Early Adversity and Postadoptive Parental Warmth', *Development and Psychopathology*, Vol. 33, No. 3, 2021, pp. 922–36. https://tinyurl.com/5fw82pth. Accessed on 12 March 2024.

mentioning the birth parents with respect and lauding their selfless love in seeking a better life for their child. Simultaneously, they should always reaffirm their status as the child's family, saying how lucky they are to have them.

One way to express this sense of belonging is by making a family book containing pictures of the parents, to which the child's picture can be added with captions. The book can be regularly updated with pictures of the entire family.

Children living with sensitive and responsive parents who are not given to volatility are likely to develop secure bonds and personalities. Following a regular routine and family rituals, like a post-dinner walk together or weekly family outings, build a sense of security for the child and parents. Celebrating occasions together—especially those linked to the child, such as their assigned birthday, the first day of school, an achievement—reinforces bonds. There is no substitute for spending quality time with the child, sans any distractions of the gadget kind, and being communicative.

Patience is the keyword. With time, the storm inside the child generally settles. If difficulties persist, then the parents should not hesitate to seek professional guidance. The child's school also needs to be made aware about the adoption and any associated psychological trauma so that the authorities handle it sensitively. Sometimes adopted children are taunted about looking different from their parents. They have to be taught how to handle such situations smartly. The matter may need to be taken up with school authorities or the parents of the bully. Requesting the cooperation of the school authorities is the way to go about it.

The age of the child and the parents at the time of adoption matters. Children who are adopted as infants form better attachments than those adopted at an older age.

Children who are older or with a past of abuse and neglect have bitter memories and have difficulty adjusting. Hearing them out in a sympathetic, non-judgemental way acts like a salve on their wounds. Constant positive engagement in parental behaviour is reassuring for them.

Younger parents tend to have more energy, while older parents are usually more sensitive and caring. Both need to be completely tuned into their child's life. The parent–child age gap decides the generation gap, which has a significant long-term impact on life and relationships.

The adjustments required in the family structure, relationships and routines are smoother if the adopted one is the first child of the family. The presence of an older birth child can complicate family life, for that child may see the adoptee as a rival and experience psychological difficulties, thus adding to the parents' stress. The sooner parents take all the children into their confidence, the better for everyone.

Moreover, they should be careful not to ignore one at the expense of the other. The message that 'we're all in this together' (a popular soft-drink jingle from the 2000s) should be repeated constantly.

Often, the curious questions of relatives, friends and neighbours about the new addition to the family might be hurtful. Parents need to prepare themselves and those around them so that their efforts at creating the family they had dreamt of get off to a good start.

Every case of adoption comes with its own set of challenges as well as rewarding experiences. For instance, children with disabilities and those with traumatic memories of past abuse often tend to act out, making the parents feel they have been rejected, and question their parenting abilities and decision to adopt. Every family relationship, be it with the self, spouse or child, can come under strain.

Such children need evaluation, intervention, special attention and care, which can be expensive. Moreover, their condition may improve only partially. Parents should take the help of therapists who treat children affected by trauma. In open adoption cases, there can be other complications. The younger the child, the easier the adjustment, otherwise the child may feel confused about the different values of adoptive and birth parents. Adoptive parents often worry about having to 'compete' with the birth family for the child's affection, and may feel accountable to the birth parents for their parenting decisions. The birth parents, on the other hand, may seem intrusive at times, especially if they try to show that they know better. The temperament of everyone involved plays a role. Having pre-established boundaries for interactions is essential.

The level of challenges tends to rise in cases of altruistic adoption, and also those where the child is from another country and culture. To bind everyone in the culture of the family, and to communicate that they are fully willing to celebrate the child's birth culture if she so desires, is not easy.

It has been observed that married adoptive parents tend to make positive adjustment better than unmarried adoptive parents do.[17] Be it a single adoption or multiple ones, the gender of the child(ren) adopted, the history of the adoptees and the adoptive family, and the availability of helping hands

---

[17]Wilson, Robin F., and W. Bradford Wilcox, 'Bringing up Baby: Adoption, Marriage, and the Best Interests of the Child', *William & Mary Bill of Rights Journal*, Vol. 14, No. 3, 2006, pp. 883–908, https://tinyurl.com/ydvejp4y. Accessed on 12 March 2024.

to raise the children—every factor influences psychological outcomes.

Adoption is a lifelong commitment, and adoption-related issues may arise at any point in the parents' or their child's lifetime. A willingness to learn about these issues and to seek support when necessary can ensure a happy family life. To the adopted children and to the adoptive parents, the family they build becomes the biggest treasure they have.

8

Forever Unbound

Some decades ago, divorce was a strict no-no. There was a stigma attached to it. A marriage was for life. In every Bollywood film, a young woman getting married was told by her parents, 'The only time you will leave your marital home will be on a bier for your final journey.'

Today, India, especially urban India, is witnessing a rise in divorce cases—not just among young couples who have wedded for love but even among those who have been in an arranged marriage for a long time.

In fact, a 2016 study based on the examination of 2011 census data brought out some revealing facts about divorce and separation in India. These can be summarized as follows:

- Although men initiate divorce more often than women, there are more instances of women remaining divorced and unmarried than men.
- Overall, more married people are opting for separation (staying apart without going through the legal process) than divorce, which can be a drain on time, money and emotional reserves. This is probably one of the reasons for India having the

lowest divorce rate in the world (around 1 per cent); the other reasons being the patriarchal hold in the Hindi-speaking states.[18]
- As of 2023, Maharashtra is the state with the highest divorce rate in India at 18.7 per cent.[19]

The social landscape has changed greatly in India's cities. There are more nuclear families with working couples. Unequal and patriarchal gender roles are changing within and outside the home. As more and more women are striving to become—and becoming—economically independent, the compulsion to stay in a toxic marriage is lessening.

People take the final step of ending their marriage when, on a regular basis, unpleasant and unacceptable aspects exceed the companionable aspects, leading to a culmination of multiple traumatic experiences.

The emotional wear and tear begins much before the divorce is actually granted. Even though divorce may spell a release from a claustrophobic marriage, it's a stressor right from the time the trauma builds up to the time a partner takes the decision to divorce, and from the painful divorce process to its aftermath.

Some opt for a separation as they want to avoid the legal process, which can be long-drawn. Some welcome

---

[18]Jacob, Suraj, and Sreeparna Chattopadhyay, 'Marriage Dissolution in India: Evidence from Census 2011', *Economic and Political Weekly*, Vol. 51, No. 33, pp. 25–7, 2016, https://tinyurl.com/4vw4xjr7. Accessed on 12 March 2024.

[19]Sarkar, Madhurima, 'States with Highest and Lowest Divorce Rates in India', *E Times*, 24 November 2023, https://tinyurl.com/5545aw8x. Accessed on 14 May 2024.

the finality offered by legal separation or divorce. In both cases, physical separation is often preceded by arguments and feelings of victimization, anger, sadness and worry about the impact on close family members. However, the physical separation should be seen as a release from daily trauma, signifying a new lease of life.

Going through a Divorce

No matter who takes the decision, its impact is felt by both partners. The degree may vary depending on the extent of social, emotional and financial dependence on the partner, support available post separation, and the magnitude of trauma suffered during the marital relationship.

While the decision to divorce is generally taken after much deliberation, the initiator spouse can still feel doubt, guilt, resentment and relief. On finding out about the decision, the non-initiator spouse, who has not had the time to process emotions, can feel a sense of disbelief and betrayal followed by thoughts of vengeance. Each of these negative emotions adds to the pre-existing stress suffered in the marital relationship.

The past cannot return physically; it haunts us emotionally and psychologically when we allow it to. Negativity can appear without warning—all it needs is a triggering comment by a relative, friend or acquaintance. It is important to recognize the warning signs and busy oneself in tasks that divert the mind—be it physical exercise, learning music, cooking, joining a group activity, or meeting new people, among others. New memories will gradually edge out old ones. What starts as a mental or physical diversion will become a regular positive habit.

To deal with self-doubt and guilt over the decision to divorce, take a pen and paper and attempt the following exercise:

- List out the problems you faced in your marriage and the steps you took to resolve them.
- Keep adding to the list to understand the extent to which you either tried to resolve a situation or surrendered to it.
- List out what else could have been done or done differently to resolve a problem.
- Now reflect on whether those methods were really feasible. Would they have achieved the desired results?

This exercise will help you understand that issues such as marital problems cannot be rectified by one person alone. This, in turn, will help you focus on the future.

Also, avoid the temptation for secrecy. Sooner or later, everyone in the family and the immediate circle is bound to know about the impending divorce. Once you tell people, you are saved the effort of making up excuses.

To create a base for future positive experiences, social support is important. Respond to people who show real concern and avoid those who try to wind you up for they are not your well-wishers. Be assertive at such times, and excuse yourself from the conversation. Women are better at dealing with the emotional aspect of divorce, in reaching out to people who comprise their support system; men not so much. The latter tend to see it as a sign of weakness, when in reality it is a sign of being human—if left too late, it could delay the healing process.

The Divorce Process and Deliberations

The divorce process is stressful in various ways. Engaging and dealing with a lawyer is an exercise in itself; their professional talk seems shorn of empathy until you grasp their role. Going to court and recounting one's trauma is painful, as are negotiations over child custody, property division and settlement of alimony.

Mediation—mutual agreement reached by representatives from both sides or a court-appointed authority—is a better alternative. It saves costs and prevents the case from dragging and prolonging emotional pain. Negotiations should always be held in the presence of experienced, sober and trustworthy elders.

Otherwise, there is no choice but to undergo the agonizing court procedure. In that event, one must develop a detached attitude towards the process and the judgement to accept reality. If that proves difficult, the resulting bitterness will impact everyone around—including the children, who will learn from the parents' behaviour.

Life after Divorce

The impact of divorce depends on multiple factors: one's age (during the separation and divorce), the number and age of the children, and whether they are in one's custody, bonding with and among children, emotional reserves and social support, financial and job stability, and the duration of the legal battle.

After the divorce, when the friends of your former spouse drop out of your life, former associates start avoiding you, and you find yourself single again and overwhelmed at having to handle so many responsibilities, just ask yourself if you are willing to exchange your present for the past. Things will fall into place.

Trust yourself and move on. Make new friends, explore new activities, keep your old faithfuls close. Spend time with your children, make simple household chores fun tasks that children can do and feel proud about. Prioritize your tasks so that you don't feel burdened. Self-time is essential to feel energized and more comfortable in your skin with every passing moment. Living with parents is also an option.

The one aspect that looms large is the question of financial security. Routine expenses, children's education, saving for a rainy day, operating on a budget—these are the new realities one must face. Be positive; it is up to you to sculpt your life the way you want.

Taking up a job or changing your present employment for something more suited to your added responsibilities could become necessary. In case of the former, you can focus on acquiring skills in an area of interest or turn a hobby into a revenue-generating exercise. It has been observed that employed mothers, even if they tend to get fatigued, are happier than unemployed ones.

Children and Significant Others

Although many people stay on in a bad marriage for the sake of their children, in reality, this is more damaging to them. Children need a loving and secure environment to grow into productive and happy individuals. It is better for them to be with a single parent in a positive atmosphere than live in an environment vitiated by either or both parents.

Children's reactions depend on various factors like their

age and bonding with siblings, proximity to the parents, exposure to marital conflict, susceptibility to biased thoughts prompted by one parent against the other, and the extent of change in their lifestyle post divorce. Remarriage of the parent with whom they are living and their relationship with the step-family also affects them.

In most cases, children stay with the mother, which adds to her responsibilities. In the post-divorce emotional roller coaster, children need adequate attention. Often, older children become defiant when a single parent, despite wanting to, is not able to devote as much time to them. If the children are much younger, they may feel a lack of guiding force in their lives.

Children of single parents are more prone to psychological changes—altered eating and sleeping patterns, depression, separation anxiety and relationship problems. Boys and girls suffer equally; how they cope differs. Generally, girls may demonstrate more internalizing behaviour (depression, guilt, withdrawal, anxiety), while boys may show externalizing behaviour (propensity for drugs and/or violence).

Some children may even blame themselves for the build-up to the divorce. Be transparent with them; give an age-appropriate explanation of the circumstances leading to the separation and reassure them that they are not at fault. Parenting requires quality time, so in whatever time you have with your children, give your 100 per cent. Engage them and engage with them, play and plan new activities with them. They will understand your position if it is explained to them, and they will empathize with you. Their company is the antidote to the blues. Be careful of transferring negative emotions on to them. Above all, steer clear of pampering and showing over-concern.

Fathers miss their children. If they have visiting rights, it is important that they keep their word about visiting the child; when that does not happen, biases get strengthened.

Parents and siblings of separated couples are also impacted, more so when they have to take emotional, social and financial care of their child/sibling and their children, if any. Besides, they may be having their own age-related issues. However, they should refrain from blaming and venting about their added responsibilities to the child, for it may send the single parent into depression.

Exploring a New Relationship

Post divorce, moving on to another relationship isn't easy. Getting involved with someone can make one feel guilty about selfishly stealing the time meant for one's children.

Any such move towards a new involvement should be made once your emotions have stabilized. It is equally important to be transparent with the children about your new relationship. Their resistance, which mainly arises from the apprehension that their parent's love and care will be divided, will abate the moment your behaviour communicates that they are still central to your life.

Besides, it is not easy to contemplate remarriage. One wonders: what if this partnership goes the same way as the previous one? Both sides need to be on the same page regarding concerns and priorities.

Before contemplating a new life with another, coming to terms with one's new reality is essential. Men in particular tend to tackle stress and boredom with alcohol, which may offer a temporary escape but only leads to further stress and depression, apart from affecting one's health and work performance. It is not the best way to project yourself. Do your thing to get back in a positive frame of mind, whether it is through physical exercise or yoga or painting. If needed, take professional help. Some move away from spiritualism, saying it did not help them; others discover spirituality as strength during a divorce crisis.

Just remember that divorce is not the end of the world—it is the end of one phase and the beginning of a new one.

9

The Modern Family

If you compare a family photograph from a generation ago with one from the present day, you are likely to see a drastic change—from several generations crowding the frame in the former to just one unit of husband, wife and children in the latter. What you are seeing is the transition from a joint family to a nuclear family, which is a reality of urban India today.

The family is the basic unit of society, the first point of human socialization. It has an important bearing on an individual's psychological make-up. The rise of the nuclear family in urban spaces has also brought changes in the psychological and mental susceptibilities of family members, posing new challenges.

A joint family is characterized by sharing of responsibilities, emotional security and coming together in times of crisis. It is also strictly hierarchical in the way rules are imposed, which can be frustrating to the younger generation.

A nuclear family is the very opposite. It is characterized by higher education levels, working couples and the financial independence of women, bound together by individualism and a sense of freedom to live the way one wants. On the flip side, there is the stress of readjustment and the absence of an 'emotional cover' in the transition from a joint to a nuclear family. The range of associated disorders in this context include adjustment disorders, depression and substance abuse. There can be an overwhelming sense of social isolation and alienation.

According to various estimates:

- The number of nuclear families in India increased from 135 million (2001) to 172 million (2011).[20]
- In urban India, 88 per cent of households comprised three–four members with no senior citizen as of 2017.[21]
- In Delhi, as of 2012, 69.5 per cent of households had only one married couple, and 17.1 per cent of households had two married couples, with a very small percentage having more than two couples.[22]

An Indian study from 2014 noted that despite being more aware of health facilities, the overall health status in nuclear families was poor as compared to joint families.[23]

---

[20]'Actually, the Nuclear Family Is on the Decline in India', *Quartz*, 1 July 2014, https://tinyurl.com/ym8k4kt3. Accessed on 12 March 2024.

[21]Terentia Consultants, 'Disintegration of the Joint Family System, Emergence of Nuclear Family', *Forbes India*, 14 December 2017, https://tinyurl.com/65stc96u. Accessed on 12 March 2024.

[22]Roy, Sidhartha, 'The Big Indian Family Breaks up, Nuclear Homes the Trend', *Hindustan Times*, 8 May 2012, https://tinyurl.com/es2fyr38. Accessed on 12 March 2024.

[23]Bansal, Sonia, et al., 'A Study to Compare Various Aspects of Members of Joint and Nuclear Family', *Journal of Evolution of Medical and Dental Sciences*, Vol. 3, No. 3, 2014, pp. 641–8, https://tinyurl.com/5xdshdsx. Accessed on 12 March 2024.

Life in Urban India

Generally, the younger generation shifts to the city for better education, job opportunities and social infrastructure. The joint family, too, sees this shift as a lifeline. By providing a taste of freedom, better jobs and finances, and a career path not only for men but also for women, the city becomes home—a base to start a marital family, a nuclear family. It also offers an escape from joint family pressures.

However, life tends to become a grind. The struggle to balance the demands of work, family, friendships and crises is emotionally sapping. Daily survival becomes the overwhelming priority. With children come new responsibilities. In some cases, couples opt not to have children.

An urban routine is like being on a treadmill constantly. Working women, who often have to work twice as hard as men to prove their worth at the workplace, shoulder comparatively more responsibilities at home as their traditional gender role demands. This can cause burnout. If the partner is immersed in his professional life and/or not supportive, a feeling of isolation arises. It's a gruelling life for men, too, for they also have to handle multiple responsibilities in the face of time restraints. Their inability to spend time with the family induces guilt in them, especially during times of special needs and occasions.

To avoid burnout, it is essential to organize one's life knowing that priorities can change with time, circumstances and experiences. Recognizing what is urgent, what can wait, and what can be avoided is important. Checklists work, but beware of checklist fatigue. The use of online transactions to pay bills, buy groceries, pay fees and EMIs, and deal with banking matters makes life easier. It just needs to be set up once.

At a time when both men and women are earning to improve the family's standing by shedding gender-assigned roles, they should share household duties as well. When men take on chores readily, it strengthens the bond between the couple and also works as a good parenting example. Otherwise, the stress generated in any one family member has the potential to disturb the entire family. If financially viable, the couple can employ someone for housework; but keep in mind that hiring and maintaining domestic staff can be stressors as well.

When both partners are working, a skewed work–life balance leaves less time for interacting meaningfully, resolving differences and discussing issues regarding parenting, disciplining and housekeeping. Plus, keeping up with the Joneses, as they say, can decrease focus on the self and one's core relationships.

When both partners are willing to listen to each other and follow up, there is an opportunity for conflict resolution. Otherwise, misunderstandings keep increasing, leading to irreparable differences. Therefore, the idea should be to minimize stress. Quit looking for perfection in household tasks, strive for a healthy work–life balance by prioritizing, be communicative with the partner, and listen without being judgemental.

The entire family should try maintaining a few rituals, such as having dinner together and spending time with each other without the distraction of gadgets. Regular outings and vacations promote sharing, caring and bonding. These can always be planned in advance.

Visible points of conflict that can snowball into discord and irreconcilable differences should be handled immediately, either mutually or with the help of trusted family and friends.

Working on stressors and revisiting life strategies with the help of elders, friends or professionals is valuable.

There may be a temptation to escape by taking substances or drugs, but that will increase stress exponentially in the long term. Adopting a healthy lifestyle, with a regular physical regimen, is the key to positivity.

Bringing up Children

Generally, a stronger financial condition and a desire to give one's child the best possible upbringing keeps nuclear families small. The emphasis is on giving children individualized attention, supporting their higher education demands, and encouraging them to pursue extracurricular activities to help them achieve their true potential. The idea is that if children observe a disciplined routine sans conflict, they learn to behave responsibly, which grooms their personality in a positive vein.

That is easier said than done. Sometimes, excessive professional and domestic demands leave little time to address the child's emotional needs, leading to maladaptive personality traits, which means that their behaviour patterns make it difficult for them to adjust when they face new or challenging circumstances in life. Added to this can be the obsessive parental focus on the child's achievements in every sphere, which accentuates the long-term negative impact on the child's personality.

Knowing the friends your child keeps and being alert to habits such as digital dependence or drugs requires time and attention. Some parents think a boarding school is the answer, but that does not work for every child, especially the sensitive and timid ones, and distances them further from the family.

Raising children in a balanced manner is one of the biggest concerns in nuclear families. Perfect parenting is an ideal, but real life, messy and emotional, gets in the way. Recognize that you need help at every stage—letting your children go to a crèche or a playschool, or having them spend time with family elders is not at all a bad idea.

Parents need to give quality time to their children. They feel wanted and important when their parents are interested in their little achievements, activities, happiness and fears. Don't make the common mistake of trying to compensate for the lack of time spent together by showering the child with material things. Children who get quality parental time generally develop a complete emotional repertoire and are socially adept. There is a greater likelihood of them being successful in life as they have a high self-esteem and better problem-solving skills. Empowering children, making them accountable, and letting them plan and handle errands are liberating.

In some nuclear families, childhood vanishes in the aggressive pursuit of parental aspirations, with very little unregimented time for the child. Excessive focus on perfection, discipline and achievement is detrimental to the child's all-round development.

Moreover, one's strength can become one's weakness as well. Children in nuclear families tend to be individualistic—sharing and caring are mostly limited to the immediate family—and run the risk developing a selfish attitude. Hence, being in touch with relatives, physically or digitally, is important. Children should be encouraged to interact with them regularly and attend social functions and festivals. All this is vital for imbibing the social values of building bonds.

The greater the social quotient, the higher the likelihood of being successful in life.

One big concern for nuclear families is the child's security, especially in view of concerns such as child abuse and neglect. Explaining the importance of staying away from strangers and teaching them to recognize a good touch from a bad touch is vital. Many couples keep an eye on the child who is alone at home or with domestic staff by means of a CCTV.

Inculcating a healthy coping mechanism in children is vital—but parents need to imbibe that first. When a parent accepts a fault without being blinded by ego, it makes the child learn that it's human to commit mistakes but good to accept and rectify them.

Elders and Other Relations

The nucleus of nuclear families is 'we and the children'. In the grind of daily responsibilities, the family gets little time to interact with friends and relatives, eroding the emotional bonds within and across generations, which are the very basis of human existence. This affects children adversely as they are unable to develop an adequate sense of community.

The lack of close relationships becomes obvious during hard times like health and financial emergencies. Normal tasks look difficult if one partner is away travelling. Nuclear families have an increased vulnerability to emotional problems, more so in the geriatric population, as evidenced during the recent Covid pandemic when families suffered for want of assistance—social, emotional and financial.

Being individualistic does not mean one is an island. In fact, it is essential to cultivate relationships with family, friends and neighbours from the beginning. It ensures that they are there for you in both happy and difficult times. Moreover, people who socialize regularly are happier (therefore less stressed) than those who don't.

A couple that insists on visiting parents during short breaks and having them stay over brings the children closer to their grandparents, strengthening the circle of life and experience. In fact, the extended nuclear family—parents of a partner staying with the couple—is fast becoming a way of life in cities. This way, the couple can look after the elderly and the elders are there for their grandchildren. However, there always has to be a sensitivity towards each other's needs and circumstances.

Looking after elders in an extended nuclear family can get tough if not handled sensitively. The nuclear family system on its own is a strong independent predictor of depression in the elderly, who feel isolated if no one has the time for them. Generally, elders are satisfied if they are listened to patiently on a regular basis, even if it is for a short while; if their medicines are in regular supply; and if their doctor's appointments are not missed.

On their part, the elders also need to comprehend the stresses of modern-day existence and empathize with the younger generation. They can find togetherness with other elderly people living in the vicinity, thus developing a vibrant community of their own.

In this new setting, recognizing limitations and maintaining boundaries helps preserve independence and bonding. The mutual understanding that everyone has their share of struggles is important for stress-free living.

Interestingly, other permutations of the family are also being worked out in cities. There are instances of joint families living as nuclear families on different floors, with one main kitchen and small pantries on each floor. Common expenses are pooled and everything else is individual. Families have their own space, and they also have each other close at hand if need be.

Clearly, the nuclear family in different forms and shapes is here to stay.

10

Life after Loss

We all yearn for someone in our lives who has our back at all times, accepts us as we are, and in whom we can confide our deepest worries and desires. Someone who also makes us see ourselves in ways we can't, encouraging us to explore our potential—it could be a close friend, a partner or a family member.

Close relationships are the safety nets that hold our lives in place, preventing us from feeling isolated. They spur personal growth and creativity, give emotional strength and a greater sense of purpose, lessen stress and thereby contribute to longevity.

Such relationships thrive on mutual respect and an understanding of the boundaries within which they work. They are strained when, due to a lack of communication or miscommunication or unarticulated expectations ('I have done so much but received nothing in return'), misunderstandings crop up. It could be just one episode or one too many, depending on the tolerance level and degree of perceived harm.

Sometimes, after a harsh statement, ego comes in the way of patching up, leading to a sense of betrayal, followed by distancing and even a break-up. It is necessary to talk it out rather than letting it fester.

Relationships are dynamic. They may not necessarily remain the same over time as circumstances keep changing. At times, despite one's best efforts, a relationship breaks. In some cases, such as when a relationship turns abusive, it is essential to break it off. Be it a misunderstanding, a traumatic break-up, or the harsh reality of death bringing a close relationship to an end, the stress generated is immense.

Grief and Bereavement

Death is a universal truth, and when someone close to us dies, it becomes a unique experience signifying a traumatic absence. The bereavement period follows, marked by grief and mourning, with specific physiological, emotional and behavioural responses. Grief is the response to loss, and mourning is the process by which people adapt to the loss. Both are greatly influenced by cultural beliefs, practices and rituals.

The Grieving Process

A grieving person usually goes through five phases—denial, anger, bargaining, sadness and acceptance. Someone could experience two phases simultaneously or not go through one of the phases; and the phases may not occur sequentially. Usually, grief starts to abate and most persons adapt to reality after six months or one year.[24]

---

[24] Mughal, Saba, et al., *Grief Reaction and Prolonged Grief Disorder*, StatPearls Publishing LLC, 14 November 2023, https://tinyurl.com/28sk6kac. Accessed on 3 May 2024.

The grieving process is shaped by a person's life experiences, such as whether the death was sudden or anticipated (due to illness or old age), one's support system, the depth of one's attachment, one's belief system, and the disruption in the quality of one's life.

The initial denial, expressed as disbelief, gives way to anger over the unfairness of having to move along an uncharted path. Anger gives a temporary sense of control over things; it could be directed against God, the system, relatives, or healthcare providers.

Anger gives way to the bargaining phase, where one promises to be a better person if the dear one were to be granted a longer lease of life. Deep inside, one knows it is futile, but the yearning is too great.

As the magnitude of the loss suffered becomes clearer, one is overcome by sadness, anxiety, detachment, emptiness and guilt. One may even start acting like the departed person. One experiences sleeplessness, lack of concentration, an inability to experience pleasure, and body aches. The impact on one's social and occupational life is tremendous.

Then comes the last stage—an intellectual and emotional acceptance of the loss, a reshaping of the self and relationships with significant others, and a reorganization and resumption of work. Readjustment to reality eventually happens between handling the deceased's belongings, dealing with financial affairs, and reaching out to other family members devastated by the loss. Some take a break to regain their professional poise. The person may keep on moving between grief and readjustment.

In case of an abrupt, violent or extremely disturbing manner of death, or where the deceased was extremely close to the bereaved, emotional breakdown verging on depression may persist even after a significant duration. The condition is called complicated grief, and it may be wise to consult a mental health professional for it.

When death occurs due to a terminal illness, relatives have time to prepare for the loss to some extent, making readjustment easier. Death in old age also brings the relief that the person's suffering is over.

The grief that follows the death of one's child, especially in teenage years or early adulthood, causes immense distress and lasts long, as the parent–child bond is deep by then. Death by suicide due to academic pressure (in part due to parental insistence) or a failed relationship is especially hard on the parents and the entire family.

Losing one's parent(s) is never easy. But the loss of old parents may be less traumatic than when parents die young. In the latter case, family members often suffer lifelong adjustment and behavioural problems, such as a higher susceptibility to substance abuse, depression, academic underachievement, and instability in future relationships.

A child facing the loss of a close family member requires the entire family's support, especially when showing worrying behavioural patterns such as sleep and appetite disturbance, irritability, destructive behaviour, withdrawal, separation anxiety, vague pains, guilt, self-harm tendencies, academic decline, and difficulty in talking about the dead person. Addressing the child's concerns and explaining the loss by using words like 'death' and 'dying' is essential; it will help the entire family.

Breaking Up with or Losing a Partner or Friend

As with other cases of loss, a break-up leads to a behavioural pattern of denial, anger, guilt, resentment, loneliness and bargaining scenarios (a vain hope that the person who exited the relationship will take the blame and want to keep the relationship going). There are simultaneous feelings of rejection and self-doubt, of wanting to be with the person as well as wanting to take revenge.

The effects of a break-up depend on which party decided to call it quits and whether it was a reasonably cordial parting or acrimonious. The break-up can, temporarily or permanently, change one's relationship with the self and others. One may lose contact with friends one knew through the estranged friend or partner.

In the case of breaking up with a partner, the sudden shift from planning a life together to the yawning absence of that person is traumatic. One feels a sense of displeasure even with the self. Also, depression may prevent one from engaging with others.

Understanding that the break-up is final is vital for recovery to begin. It has to be a complete break with the person, which means the cessation of all communication. Remember, time is a great healer. Also, do not lose faith in people and relationships. It takes strength of character to move on from a relationship that had earlier been one's strength.

Whether and when to enter into a new relationship is another important question. It would be prudent to wait for the grief to be over before exploring a new relationship, as impulsive decisions taken during emotional turmoil can backfire.

The psychological and emotional stress that follows the

death of a close friend can be as bad as, or worse than, that caused by the death of a family member. However, society doesn't place friendship at the same level as family ties. Due to the inadequacy of social support, the grieving one may feel alone in their grief. That bereavement should not be belittled.

Pain of Loss: Factors Impacting the Magnitude of Agony

Although susceptibility to stress differs from person to person, it is safe to say that there are aggravating and mitigating factors that interact in a complex manner to determine stress intensity:

- Stress depends on the duration of affection and dependency in a relationship—the death of a spouse or a child is among the most stressful.
- A sudden and unexpected death is more traumatic than one that is anticipated, for in the latter, reality sets in early.
- A number of bereavements faced in a short duration can cause significant stress, as happened during Covid-19 in many households, leaving the survivors with intense emotional turmoil.
- Doing everything possible during treatment prior to death reduces stress. The inability to help a person change harmful lifestyle choices (drug consumption, lack of exercise and diet control, etc.) may be guilt-inducing.
- The aftermath of death, such as being distanced from the departed one's friend circle, can be painful.

- Any unfinished financial deal adds to prevailing stress.
- Higher educational levels and emotional reserves, close emotional bonds, a steady job and a good state of health can reduce stress. Generally, women suffer more intense and longer-lasting psychological trauma than men. Being agreeable, conscientious, emotionally stable and open to experience creates resilience against stress.
- Youngsters can muster more social support but are psychologically less mature. Older people may have the maturity but lack adequate social support. Those at the end of the age spectrum suffer more.
- The greatest impact occurs soon after and around the anniversary of the event.
- Generally, suffering decreases with the passage of time. As they say, 'Time is a great healer.'
- Greater suffering is experienced if one is burdened with the roles and responsibilities of the departed.

Dealing with Grief

Grief is a highly personal experience. There is no right or wrong way to grieve. So let yourself feel the emotions without embarrassment—it's okay to cry, be sad, or yell at the heavens. Crying doesn't mean you are weak, and grief doesn't mean being serious all the time; it's natural to have moments of lightness even during grief. Instead of putting on a brave face for the sake of family and friends, showing one's true feelings is more helpful.

Healing cannot be forced. Mourning depends on factors like personality profile, resilience, lived experiences, faith, and what loss means to the person in question. Pain that is buried deep inside will surface eventually, so it's better to actively deal with grief to move on.

There are many positive coping mechanisms—socialization, adaptation, distraction, altruism, forgiveness, journal writing, art and pet therapy, among others.

Viewing death as an integral part of life helps. Use the strengths you possess to cope. Self-care activities, such as proper nutrition, ample sleep, meditation and listening to soothing music, are important. Drifting towards alcohol or drugs is counterproductive.

Grief associated with some circumstances is not acknowledged by society, such as having an abortion or the death of a pet, lover or ex-partner. This is called disenfranchised grief, where no formal grief pattern and social support may be available. The grieving individual may have to suffer alone. It is important to mourn, so one must be assertive and seek support at least from those who are empathetic.

Those who believe in the mourning traditions of various religions can seek solace in praying, chanting, reciting mantras, listening to hymns, meditating, or going to a place of worship. In the case of any doubts, discussion with a trusted person or respected practitioner is advised.

The death of someone close is bound to make one aware of one's own mortality. But that doesn't mean that one's end is arriving *now*, so avoid impulsive actions like giving away one's essential assets or spending recklessly. Any minor change in bodily function may cause concern but shouldn't be considered anything serious. If it's a new symptom, visiting a doctor may be warranted but panic is not.

When it is unclear whether one did what was best for the person who died, the result is guilt. At such a juncture, the family should act in unison, supporting each other rather than accusing each other of any act(s) of omission or commission. This was witnessed during the pandemic, when people lost their kin despite their best intentions and efforts, as the larger circumstances were beyond their control. Better to forgive yourself and others rather than blame everyone around you. Most importantly, give yourself time to heal.

There is a persistent anxiety about losing one's connection with the deceased and a guilt associated with 'feeling better' (or allowing a new person into one's life). That doesn't mean that the person one has lost is being forgotten; it just means that one has acknowledged reality. Till the emotional turmoil eases, try not to associate with places, people or activities that have the power to trigger distress.

Be prepared to have moments of distress on anniversaries and festive occasions, and guard against being constantly overwhelmed by them. Be vigilant enough to consciously break the chain of sad thoughts by engaging in some pre-decided mental or physical activity. Keep trusted ones close; their support can be invaluable. Remember that you have a precious pact with life and should honour it.

However, when the grief is of a higher intensity or long duration, making life difficult for oneself or close ones, it is time to consult a mental health professional.

11

The Empty Nest Syndrome

When most middle-class couples in urban India start a family, they are determined to provide the best of opportunities to their children. When that aspiration becomes a reality, and the child has to leave home for further studies or a job in another city or country, the parents' happiness and pride are tinged with apprehension.

Marriage is another significant reason for children moving away. Further reasons for relocation could be related to altercations within the family or a desire by either of or both parties to shirk responsibilities and retain independence. A lack of space due to living in a small house that is unable to accommodate all the members of the family may also result in separation.

The reduction of one member from a nuclear family that is already small (with one or two children) has a greater emotional impact on family members, especially the parents. Fresh capacities and strengths need to be developed to readjust to the new reality.

Parents need to understand that it's okay to feel emotionally upset at this stage in life, and there is no need to feel guilty about it either. They do realize that children moving out to achieve higher goals is a fact of life and something to be proud of. But they also know that it's a watershed moment—the young one leaving the nest to take flight.

The young one's departure is followed by a sense of loss of purpose, an identity crisis, and even a feeling of rejection, for it seems as if the parental role is over. Despite life proceeding as it always did, with the presence of other relatives and ongoing social activities, parents feel hollow inside, as if something vital is missing.

Attachment is often accompanied with emotional dependency, and separation with a stressful vacuum. Some parents are impacted for a short period, some for much longer. For some, the impact can even be lifelong. Either parent or both may experience loneliness, anxiety and depression. The need for medication may increase.

Those who are more vulnerable to suffering in such circumstances include parents who:

- are old and have medical or psychiatric illnesses;
- are dependent on the child(ren) for finances, daily activities, hospital visits or technology-related issues;
- have an unsatisfactory or unstable marital life;
- are single and have no other social support except the child(ren);
- are experiencing other painful life events simultaneously, like losing a loved one or the start of an illness;
- have low self-worth and see change as stressful, not challenging or refreshing;
- are focussed full-time on parenting and do not expand their own horizons;
- invest all their emotional energies in the excessive care and pampering of their child; and

- have perceived all the other milestones in the child's life—going to school, having their first romantic crush—as painful.

Mothers, including those who are working professionals, tend to be impacted more intensely as they are usually more involved in the child's life at every stage. Homemakers are more troubled, for it seems to them that their primary role is over. Feeling a lack of self-worth, they are left unsure about how to proceed.

The empty nest syndrome is a term given to the changes and difficulties experienced by parents when their children move out of home. Sometimes, even when a younger child is living with the family, the mother especially may feel grief when the older, emotionally closest child relocates for studies or a job, or after marriage. For instance, after the marriage of a daughter closest to her (being the mother's strongest emotional and practical support), she may go into depression, for it may seem as if she has no one to share her intimate thoughts and feelings with, or to help her reach decisions.

If the child is relocating for studies, the primary causes for worry are whether the child will:

- be adequately prepared to live independently;
- maintain the emotional connection and call regularly;
- be able to cope with the challenges of daily living and circumstances including an illness;
- manage finances sensibly;
- fall into bad company or habits like substance abuse;
- get into a relationship;
- obey parental wishes or turn rebel; and
- return or settle in another city.

The parents' control over the child's life, something that had been a given for many years, suddenly slips, causing frustration. What if the young one is leading a life that does not match their expectations? That is their biggest worry.

Realize that you're not losing the child who is leaving the parental home to pursue studies or a job. It's a sign that you did everything right. If you trust your parenting skills, then surely learning to cope in a new setting will build the child's character.

New habits should not be seen as negative; they are a response to a new environment and a new awareness of the world. But if you sense something disturbing, then it's better to talk about it and get a response.

However, do not transfer your anxiety by trying to micromanage the youngster's life from a distance. It will backfire. It may result in extreme passivity or rebellion, thus impeding the organic growth of the child's personality and academic, professional or marital life. Eventually, both child and parents suffer.

A balance is needed between being in the know and over-involvement. For instance, it is sensible to call at a mutually-agreed-upon time. However, if it turns out that the youngster is in a vulnerable situation, the parents have every right to intervene.

Meanwhile, the parents should try to bring their lives back on an even keel. Wallowing in sadness attracts negativity easily. Divert your mind by engaging in some activity, physical, mental or social. Develop new interests, which will create a new social circle for you as well. There are abundant worlds to be explored online related to your interests, be it music, spiritualism, wildlife or sport. You could keep a journal, join a book club, or rekindle old friendships, as most of your peers would be going through a similar phase. It might be interesting to start a parents' support group with those friends. Bring alive the bucket list that had been cast aside in the hurly-burly of bringing up children. Employment or re-employment are options, as is volunteer work. Self-care activities are also rewarding.

Do not ignore your health. Learn to do the things your child did to manage your medical condition, otherwise the condition may become uncontrollable, creating stress for yourself and the child, who will be ridden with guilt.

With the departure of the young one, whose presence might have prevented marital issues from snowballing, old and new marital issues can surface, sometimes leading to divorce after decades of being together. Consequently, the entire family suffers, the child living at a distance more so.

The spouses may react differently to the reality that the child has left the parental home. They can drift apart or they can be sensitive to each other's angularities and problems by keeping communication lines open and readjusting to new realities.

Remember that for the child, who may be away from home for the first time, living alone is not easy either. Though happy to start a new chapter of life, the youngster may simultaneously be homesick.

If there is anything constant in life, it is change. Roles and responsibilities become different with age. It is not that children never left home for their vocations back in the day, but families used to be larger and the world was not the global village that it is at present. Relocating for positive purposes should be taken as a sign of growth. Besides, unlike in the past, technology keeps us connected in a way we never could have imagined. Ultimately, what today's parents want to be sure of is the child's emotional support.

All children don't move out for pleasant reasons. A smaller house unable to accommodate many people, regular altercations (between parents and children, among siblings, or between mother-in-law and daughter-in-law), fear of handling the responsibility of old and ailing parents, a marriage against the parents' wishes—all these could be triggers for some to move out.

Sometimes, parents themselves tell the child to move out for the sake of preserving peace in the family, or because of their awareness that children should be able to lead their lives the way they want.

Parents need to understand that how the child turns out in later years is a reflection of their rearing. Hence, their own education, with some dos and don'ts, needs to start from the time the child is born:

- Avoid being an overprotective and over-involved parent. It stunts everyone's growth—yours as well as the child's.
- Don't be too strict or too indulgent; a balanced upbringing equips the child the best.
- Don't play favourites with your children. Be fair in dealings with siblings; address sibling rivalry by encouraging discussion and complimenting both sides for their contributions.
- Give every family member a say in family matters. This will help the young feel included.
- Emphasize the value of a good education in the classroom and outside as well. This would mean not just acquiring intellectual skills, but also an experiential knowledge of rights, responsibilities,

freedom and its limits, and help cultivate emotional understanding and ethical behaviour.

It is these qualities that will always keep the child and parents connected and prepared to face new challenges with a positive mindset.

When a child leaves the parental home for studies or for a job, the element of sadness that parents feel often goes unacknowledged, as the move is seen as something natural and progressive. Sometimes, the feeling of sadness can lead to depression and anxiety, or the flaring up of physical illnesses.

Generally, this life event tends to coincide with other stressful life events, like menopause or the start of an illness, making it more difficult to adapt to the new reality. This is all the more reason to ensure that the parent-child relationship evolves in a new direction, while keeping the basic emotional connection intact.

The fact is that all of us know about the human life cycle, that time waits for no one. Perhaps it is essential to internalize this universal truth in our personal lives so we can craft our familial relationships with care from the very beginning. It is the least that parents can do—after all, they were children once, and their children will be parents someday.

12

Solo Parenting

Being a single mother is twice the work, twice the stress, and twice the tears but also twice the hugs, twice the love, and twice the pride.

—Unknown

The number of families headed by lone mothers is on the increase in India. According to a report by UN Women, *Progress of the World's Women 2019–2020: Families in a Changing World*, single-parent families comprise 8 per cent of all Indian households, of which 4.5 per cent (about 13 million) families are headed by single mothers. Apart from this, roughly 32 million single mothers stay with extended family, according to the report.[25]

Death, separation and single-woman births are the leading reason for single-parent families.[26] According to the

---

[25] UN Women, *Progress of the World's Women 2019–2020: Families in a Changing World*, 2019, https://tinyurl.com/2kht8afe. Accessed on 12 March 2024.

[26] Bhat, Nasir Ahamd, and R.R. Patil, 'Single Parenthood Families and Their Impact on Children in India', *Delhi Psychiatry Journal*, Vol. 22,

UN Women report, the number of divorcees in India have doubled in the past two decades, with the largest proportion occurring in urban areas.[27] Other reasons for single parenting could be the partner's demise, single-person adoption, and a single woman's decision to have a child. A situation where one partner lives in another city or country is almost similar to that of single parenting.

Single or lone parenting includes:

- singular parenting, when only one parent takes care of the child;
- cooperative parenting, when separated parents correspond with each other about how to raise the child; and
- parallel parenting, when separated parents don't talk to each other about the child; the child is shifted between parents for specific time periods.

Challenges of Single Parenting

Single parenting comes with its own challenges. Taking on both gender roles and experiencing greater autonomy can be seen as a positive. The pluses include better parenting, a strong parent–child bond and shared responsibilities, leading to a blurring of gender roles.

To accomplish all this by fulfilling both gender roles and being solely responsible for the family's emotional

---

No. 1, 2019, pp. 161–5, https://tinyurl.com/4dyusnuy. Accessed on 26 April 2024.

[27]UN Women, *Progress of the World's Women 2019–2020: Families in a Changing World*, 2019, https://tinyurl.com/wdwnk3zd. Accessed on 12 March 2024.

and material health can put enormous stress on the single parent. Often, lone-parent families (especially lone-mother families) have limited access to social, emotional and financial resources. The estimates derived from the data on household size and composition from the 2009–10 employment survey, when combined with *World Population Prospects: The 2017 Revision*, yield some troubling conclusions.[28] These are:

- Poverty rates of single-mother households with children up to the age of six or younger are higher than those of two-parent households in India.
- Poverty rate of lone-mother households is 38 per cent, in comparison to 22.6 per cent for dual-parent households.

Several factors affect the stress level. The younger the single parent and children, the greater the likelihood of stress. The financial condition, extent of social support, bonding among siblings, and the parent's educational background and employment status also matter. Moreover, the parent's personality and mental health affect the way they handle the stress of life events such as a difficult divorce, abandonment or the painful death of a partner.

Parental separation impacts the children in various ways. Young children often feel abandoned and confused, and have trouble coping. In grown-up children, acceptance of divorce may be accompanied with distrust for both parents, feelings of shame, guilt and resentment, difficulties in academic

---

[28]Pandit, Ambika, 'Single Mothers Head 4.5% of All Indian Households', *The Times of India*, 8 July 2019, https://tinyurl.com/3fav3mwv. Accessed on 12 March 2024.

performance, and problems in emotional growth that could impact their ability to form and sustain relationships.

Constant comparison with children living with both parents is stressful, not just for the child but for the single parent as well, with the latter wondering if enough is being done to care for the young. Sometimes, young children's constant questions about the absent parent and inability to grasp explanations can put immense pressure on the single parent, especially if the separation was traumatic. Fatigue sets in, leading to scolding and self-guilt. At times, single parents do what two-parent families also do to avoid uncomfortable questions—point the child towards the screen.

The parent and the extended family should patiently give an age-appropriate explanation, making it clear that neither was the decision to separate taken lightly, nor were the children responsible for it. Children are deeply understanding, and if patient and transparent discussions are accompanied with productive activities that engage their minds, the results will be positive.

Moreover, nothing can equal spending quality time with the children, helping them deal with their emotions. It helps everyone overcome trauma and focus on the present. If the child feels loved and secure, over time, the questioning and restlessness regarding the other parent tends to decrease. It helps if close relatives form a circle of love around the youngsters, encouraging them to come out of their shell.

Parenting during the divorce process or soon after separation is a fraught task as the parent is dealing with their own demons as well. Most of the time, such life-altering decisions are taken after much thought. Hence, looking back with regret only detracts from positive parenting. Remaining in the same neighbourhood and school is better for the child's immediate adjustment but not easy practically.

If the single parent is living with the children's grandparents, the latter should refrain from raking up the past and blaming one or the other parent for the state of affairs. Using the children to settle personal scores is counterproductive. Sometimes, the extended family along with the single parent make the meeting between the children and the absent parent uncordial. All it does is create an atmosphere of mistrust and resentment, which is harmful for everyone.

Remember, children are shaped by the context in which rearing takes place. Avoid compensating for the unsettling environment following the separation by providing material gifts. Understand the fine line between concern and over-concern. The latter will only hamper their long-term development.

Lone parents have to handle everything from managing the day-to-day running of the household and seeing to the nurturing and education of the children, to handling a job and finances and keeping the family's social support alive. Each domain competes for time, energy and effort, and that can be a stressor in itself.

Younger children crave affection, and the parent may feel guilty about not being able to be there for important occasions like school functions, or just playing and bonding with the children. As opposed to two-parent families, children from single-parent families are at a higher risk of developing excessive internalized and externalized negative behaviours. In the former, excessive emotional control manifests as depression, withdrawal, inhibition, self-esteem problems and anxiety. The latter is marked by an absence of emotional control, leading to impulsive and aggressive behaviour.[29]

Children are more at risk of developing negative behaviours, be it lagging behind in academics, drug use, taking to crime or age-inappropriate sexual behaviour, all of which impacts their mental and physical health. With adolescents, there is also the anxiety about them falling under negative influences outside the home. On the other hand, in some cases, the parent–child bond may be so strong that they suffer from separation anxiety.

Parenting is not an easy task under any circumstance, more so for a single parent. The dilemma of how and how much to discipline is the issue. If the household is run according to unambiguous rules, with every member clear about what he or she has to do, children are bound to feel settled. It is important to be proportionate in disciplining unacceptable behaviour. Losing privileges often makes children realize the error of their ways. Likewise, good behaviour should be appreciated and rewarded proportionately.

The trick is to create a routine that draws children in, makes them feel in control and responsible. Assign age-appropriate tasks at home or outside (tidying up rooms, buying milk, and so on). Once in a while, say, after exams, punctuate the daily routine with a 'no rules, all fun' day. Be receptive to their likes and dislikes, listen to them in a

---

[29]Daryanani, Issar, et al., 'Single Mother Parenting and Adolescent Psychopathology', *Journal of Abnormal Child Psychology*, Vol. 44, No. 7, 2016, pp. 1411–23, https://tinyurl.com/4ssmprb8. Accessed on 12 March 2024; Chavda, Kersi, and Vinyas Nisarga, 'Single Parenting: Impact on Child's Development', *Journal of Indian Association for Child and Adolescent Mental Health*, Vol. 19, No. 1, 2023, pp. 14–20, https://tinyurl.com/2p8bxkz3. Accessed on 12 March 2024.

non-judgemental way, and they will confide in you. Most of all, let them know that your love for them is unconditional. Simultaneously, keep an eye on their behaviour, tackling any issue the moment it arises. Children who spend quality time with a parent are more likely to have a well-adjusted personality. A parent who is not overly dependent on gadgets is a positive influence.

For a single parent who wears multiple hats, it is all the more important to attempt a balance between professional and personal life. If frustrated about something, explain to the children that the negative emotions have nothing to do with them. Share age-appropriate issues with them—this way, children will also feel free to express themselves. Comparing one's life with that of the estranged partner is best avoided.

If the children are young, the parent has little time for the self. However, when children start taking on responsibilities and develop confidence with age, a parent may get some time and personal space.

It is important for a single-parent family to have social support. The presence of extended family members, such as grandparents and friends who can step in to help, is crucial. The grandparent–grandchild bond is special, but there should be an awareness of the basic ground rules of parenting. If there is a difference of opinion between the grandparents and single parent, it should be sorted out when the children are not around.

Over-investing time and energy on children can suffocate lives. From the beginning, single parents must prioritize a healthy lifestyle to remain active and retain contact with the social circle that cushions them against loneliness. A word of advice: pick up the phone and talk to friends; steal an hour or so during the weekend. Be positive and think of finding solutions to problems, rather than wallowing in self-pity. Joining a support group is an option.

Parents who immerse themselves in their children's lives often feel betrayed if youngsters want to follow their hearts. This happens especially when the parents are older and their expectations are greater. The child's rebelliousness or difference of opinion is generally more difficult to handle in mother–son and father–daughter relationships.

In father–daughter and mother–son relationships, adolescence issues like hormonal changes, relationship woes, gadget dependence and even drug abuse may crop up more. Adolescents prefer to talk to their own gender. Instead of confiding in the parent, they may take the Internet as their guide or look for advice from people who may not be reliable and rather dangerous at times. That is why it is better to raise the child in an environment where anything can be shared unhesitatingly. An attempt can then be made to find a solution, but this requires empathy and non-judgemental listening.

Managing the household and fulfilling the children's educational requirements on a single income is the toughest aspect. Try to live within your means, distinguishing between need and luxury and discussing it with the children. If a computer is needed, for instance, rather than going for the latest model, buy an older one which is perfect for the children's purpose, telling them that by doing so they are doing their bit for the planet in an age of mindless technological obsolescence. Smart explanations help. They generally understand that love does not mean granting their every wish. Financial support for educational purposes from one's support circle can also be helpful.

Financial independence comes from a job, which is an

important source of self-worth and social connections as well. It can create stress, too—more so for a single parent juggling too many responsibilities. On the whole, it has been observed that although employed single mothers feel more fatigue, they are happier than those who are unemployed.

The other significant issue of getting into a new relationship is thorny, for any transition of this kind generates stress and impacts parenting. The decision depends on many considerations, like the children's experiences with the separated parent, their age and current mental state, the personality of the future partner, and the availability of family support.

Though a difficult topic to bring up with children, especially when they are very young, it is better to discuss it openly with them and the prospective partner during the courtship period. Communicate to the children that their centrality in your life will not change. Approach the extended family or a counsellor to talk to the children about the prospective relationship. Don't be impatient; the decision can go either way. Similarly, you need to weigh your options if the prospective partner doesn't understand your dilemma.

Ultimately, it is up to you whether you want to see the glass as half empty or half full. Single parenthood can be tough, but it can be equally rewarding as well.

13

Health Is the True Wealth

On the one hand, advances in medicine have provided a cure for diseases considered fatal earlier or helped us manage them better. On the other hand, lifestyle diseases are reaching almost epidemic proportions in India, especially in cities and towns, manifesting in younger age groups as well.[30] Moreover, while many an infective disease has been brought under control, the recent pandemic, which has altered our lives in so many ways, is proof that there will always be new diseases to study and control.

It is a fact that people with lifestyle issues and weaker immunity suffer more severely, and that it is urban Indians who have more lifestyle issues. The pandemic underscored the importance of maintaining the delicate balance within the body—a reality that many urban Indians had forgotten in the bustle of city life, thinking that the body would take care of itself.

How can that be possible with a largely sedentary lifestyle, unhealthy dietary habits, sleep deprivation, lack of exercise due

---

[30]'Lifestyle Diseases in India', *Press Information Bureau*, 31 July 2018, https://tinyurl.com/3wm4j9xk. Accessed on 12 March 2024.

to long working hours, busy schedules and long travel times to and from the workplace? Let's not forget the stress that goes with this, all of which weakens the body's immunity, leaving it vulnerable to disease. City life is exhilarating, no doubt, provided one takes care of one's overall health.

Illness requires fresh adjustment, both in body and mind. Issues concerning the illness, its treatment, the personality and resilience of the patient and caregivers, finances and available social support, individually or collectively, have the potential to generate stress, affecting not just the patient but family and friends as well.

The etymological meaning of the word 'disease' is 'not at ease'. Whether a person has an acute or severe disease or chronic condition(s), it demands financial resources, lifestyle changes and several restrictions. All in all, the effort required generates stress.

There are three dimensions to disease: predisposition, precipitating factors and perpetuating factors. There is not much that can be done with genetic predisposition, but many precipitating and perpetuating factors like diet and lifestyle are alterable. If an illness is past the preventive stage, there is at least the possibility of containment after it has crossed the intense phase.

In case of disorders with a strong family history (like diabetes and hypertension), lifestyle changes can even stop or delay their onset. Yes, it is difficult to break one's inertia, but not impossible—people just need changes in sleep and screen time, diet, exercise and rejuvenation.[31]

---

[31]Nicoll, Rachel, and Michael Y. Henein, 'Hypertension and Lifestyle Modification: How Useful Are the Guidelines?', *British Journal of General Practice*, Vol. 60, No. 581, 2010, pp. 879–80, https://tinyurl.com/5h7yujkm. Accessed on 12 March 2024.

Also, there's a general notion that taking medication is a sign of weakness. One needs to go by hard facts, and if the treatment needs medication, then go with medicine for the prescribed period.

The idea of regular medical check-ups has still not become a routine part of our daily lives. We often go to the doctor only when a problem crops up, which leads to unpleasant consequences at times.

When a person is diagnosed with a serious disease all of a sudden, it comes as a shock to the entire family and circle of close friends. The stress is enormous. It is very important for family and friends to provide vital support to the person struggling with illness and treatment, and to each other as well. Whether a chronic or acute condition, the attitude of family members plays an important role. For example, in the case of a chronic condition like diabetes, at least until the person in question makes a lifestyle change successfully, other family members could decide to not keep sweets in the house, indulging their own desires outside. Similarly, for an acute condition like an infectious disease, family members could choose to be strict about the hygiene protocol.

Some illnesses like HIV have a stigma attached to them, while news about one being diagnosed with a disease like cancer can traumatize the entire family. Many families prefer to keep the disease and treatment a secret. However, sharing the news with close friends and relatives leads to sharing of pain, and keeps the person connected to the much-needed warmth of supportive and empathetic relatives. To break the news takes much courage, but to hide one's condition saps one of energy that can be used positively.

In India, many families debate whether they should tell the patients about the severity and nature of their illness.

Most of the time, there is a presumption that they will not be able to take the bad news. In reality, most patients are well aware of their situation; it is just that they have not expressed it. The family should understand that.

The Painful Treatment Process

At first, there is the stress that comes upon realizing that you or your dear one is seriously ill. Then comes the stressful task of finding the right doctor. The extent of specialization often leads to confusion about whom to consult. Instead of trying to scout for names online, it is better to consult a general physician in your area who can then guide you. It is a good idea to ask close relatives and friends as well.

Over time, the doctor–patient relationship has undergone some change that can cause additional stress. From a paternalistic, trustful relationship, it has now become more of a service-provider–client relationship. From the patient's end, waning trust and high expectations, such as believing that they own the doctor's time and services because of the fee being paid, create problems; at the doctor's end, disappearing sympathy, time constraints and unapproachability become problematic.

Providing the patient information based on facts is the doctor's brief. Some are diplomatic, some straightforward, some explain things in detail, and others partially. One may feel that the doctor in question is abrasive, but if the given facts answer one's queries, it is preferable to having a doctor who has winning ways.

Many go for a second, third or fourth opinion. Some try scientifically unestablished treatments, but when their condition deteriorates, the patients return to the doctor.

Taking the expert's help on time not only reduces suffering but saves finances too. Treatment guidelines are framed after years of research, so it is better to follow the doctor's advice and not self-medicate or follow unresearched or unproven therapies. Once that level of trust is established, the patient's stress levels reduce.

A Predisposition to Indisposition

The personality and mental make-up of the patient and family members have a lot to do with the level of stress experienced. The burden felt is inversely proportional to one's resilience—to some, even short-term distress is unbearable, while others take even chronic illnesses in their stride.

To anxious people, even a minor indisposition seems a big disease. They are prone to taking medication for the slightest distress while simultaneously being worried about the medication's side effects, and also the financial pressure and consequences of the illness.

Those who suffer from anxiety should realize the fact and consult a mental health expert to address it because anxiety is life-limiting and often becomes an impediment to the pursuit of a healthy social and/or occupational life. Excessive worrying may require medication and counselling.

People who are quick to blame themselves often take illness as a personal failure and are filled with guilt, wondering where they went wrong. If the disease is severe, worriers go into a loop of endless questions—'Why me? What have I done wrong? Haven't I always been helpful to others?' and so on. The fact is that that the human body is like a machine—it works well initially but if not maintained properly, it deteriorates, more so when it has been handled rashly, which may lead to disease if not attended to in time. One should see disease for what it is instead of as a punishment.

Illnesses and treatment have a factual basis, and it is better to know from the doctor what to expect during the treatment and the lifestyle changes that may be needed. Once that trust is established, one should stop worrying. It not only impacts the severity of the illness but delays recovery as well. Sometimes, people who are impatient by nature and expect a fast recovery change therapies frequently. This is counterproductive and only delays proper treatment.

Like everything else in nature, the human body goes through its cycle of growth and decline. Some people live in denial, thinking nothing can happen to them, and leave the treatment or only take it partially. Sooner or later, any untreated illness will have painful consequences. Accepting the illness, following the doctor's advice, making all efforts for recovery, and adhering to the prescribed regimen will greatly reduce the stress of the patient and caregivers.

In today's times, worriers have a field day trawling the Internet for any details of the illness that is affecting them or their family members. Their focus is drawn to the negative aspects, increasing their anxieties all the more, be it the long-term consequences of the illness or side effects of the medication.

Often, patients who go for a medical consultation end up telling the doctor what they think they are suffering from, on the basis of the information they have found on the Internet, instead of waiting for the expert to tell them. Most of the time, the information gathered is anxiety-inducing and creates distrust in the doctor–patient relationship. Stress aggravates the illness, and the illness leads to escalation of stress. The medical fraternity has a term for this completely avoidable tendency—IDIOT, or Internet derived information obstructing treatment.

A better course is to write down one's doubts and questions and ask the doctor to clarify them. But remember, the doctor provides facts, which may or may not be in sync with your emotions or expectations.

From the initial visits to the doctor and specialist, followed by investigations, to the treatment and post-treatment life, the financial pressure is quite high up in the minds of families. The sorry state of most public health infrastructure in the country means that most people have no option but to visit private institutions. At times, the costs can be crippling for a middle-class family. It is commonly said that the treatment for a serious illness can deplete one's lifetime savings rapidly. Overall, getting treated 'satisfactorily' has become a mind-boggling exercise.

This is one reason why it is sensible to invest in a medical insurance policy as soon as possible, the limits of which can be increased steadily. Saving for unexpected expenses is necessary. Apart from this, the best insurance is to try and maintain a balanced lifestyle to the extent possible.

Making everything doubly difficult is the emotional stress a family goes through when a member falls seriously ill. If it is a nuclear family, it is important to have a close circle of friends and relatives who can be counted upon at all times. These days, there are support groups online and offline, and it is sensible to explore the options their members suggest to get an idea of how the stress of similar circumstances was handled by them.

At times, the illness of a family member to whom one's attachment is not very strong or has declined over time, for example an elder or a child with chronic illness or a relative with a drug dependence, may seem a burden. However, such circumstances are not unique to one family; they are part of our social reality. It is better to find a way to do one's duty by cultivating a certain amount of detachment. It helps to have people with whom one can give vent to one's feelings. That way, some of the stress eases.

It is important to understand that the rhythm of present-day urban life is such that it is exhilarating and stressful at the same time. The attempt should be to keep away from excess and strive for a balanced lifestyle that includes a physical and de-stressing regimen so that one can stay in the zone of prevention. There are many options available. Choose the physical regimen you like, whether it is walking, running or going to the gym, and/or yoga and meditation. Maintain a healthy diet schedule and hygiene. Have a good social circle of friends with whom you can relax and laugh or vent your feelings. Be assertive in relationships to avoid stress. Also, have regular medical check-ups after a certain age, say 40. Don't do these things to tick a box. Do these to change the quality of your life so that you get the benefit of a healthy existence.

Remember, it's your health we are talking about here. Do you want to take it lightly?

14

Money, Money, Money...

*A wise man should have money
in his head, but not in his heart.*

—Jonathan Swift

There was a time when the word 'priceless'—meaning something whose worth cannot be measured by money alone—was used frequently. Today, money has become the sole measure of the worth of practically everything. It exemplifies success, power, prestige and influence. Making money has become almost a religion.

This fundamental shift is creating its own set of dilemmas and pressures in India's urban landscape. The stress caused by a lack of financial resources has always been familiar to large sections of our society, but the pressures triggered by the ceaseless quest of money in an aspirational society are new and unsettling.

When Wants Become Needs

Everyone understands that money is essential for fulfilling the needs of day-to-day life, namely food, clothing, shelter, education and recreation, in sync with one's socio-economic background. The lack of financial resources for any one of these aspects can be crippling. The idea of saving for a rainy day, too, is a familiar concept for Indians. After the basic needs are met, people look towards bettering their lives through better education, better housing and going on several holidays in a year, among other things.

Before one realizes, wants become needs—that high-end car, or cell phone, or refrigerator... Life is lived in instalments—EMIs. There is a constant pressure to earn more, especially in light of inflation. Monetary requirements of households keep spiralling.

Those engaged in entrepreneurial activities face similar challenges of an ever-growing need for finances. Ironically, the hours of work keep extending, leaving little time for the family or oneself, not to mention the adverse impact this has on one's health. On top of that, one often feels a sense of guilt at not being able to provide enough for the family, compared to many others. Exhaustion overwhelms the person.

The growing gap between what one perceives as unmet needs and income becomes a constant source of worry, especially if one has family responsibilities and a history of financial anxiety. The stress may become chronic. Poor financial and mental health are directly related, one leading to the other. The vicious cycle continues.

If one is facing a dip in monetary fortunes after having experienced an affluent phase, the trauma is worse, as it is difficult to let go of luxurious habits. There can be a real lack of finances, and there can also be a feeling of a lack of financial well-being in comparison with others. Both situations can lead to discontentment and disagreements with family, friends, employees or customers.

The first step to avoiding the stress of such situations is to know where you stand and what your dreams are. The state of your finances and your responsibilities are your reality, where you stand. Your dreams are your aim, and you need to make a plan for accomplishing material comforts in stages, without giving yourself undue strain. Remember, life is not a sprint, nor is it just about a certain lifestyle; it is a gift to you. Live your life at your pace.

Living on a budget is not something alien to Indians; generations have lived like that. A budget is a spending plan that takes into account both current and future income and expenses. It keeps a check on spending, ensures savings, helps in figuring long-term financial goals, and helps avoid credit card debt. You may surprise yourself by your ability to stay on the budget track.

Distinguishing between need and want is purely a matter of common sense. For instance, gadgets that are essential to one's work are a need. Making optimal use of resources is something that all Indians have imbibed from earlier generations—using gadgets till they last and choosing repair over replacement by the 'latest' model saves money. A vehicle may be necessary for work, but it need not be a luxury model.

Many families develop the habit of prudent shopping, such as buying necessities in bulk. Saving small amounts through discretionary spending can yield a nice nest egg. If the whole family is invested in budgeting, things go far smoother.

Of course, this is easier said than done. Often, negative emotions dominate—such is the pull of an aspirational lifestyle. Credit card spending may become an addiction, putting people in a tight spot again and again. Anxiety and depression are common outcomes.

When savings are exhausted, loans mount and lenders start threatening, or if there are major expenses ahead, the stress is palpable. In some cases, as published frequently in newspapers, individuals caught in a debt trap end their lives, or even take to crime to fuel their aspirations.

When such situations occur, evasion may seem the only way out. Explaining the real financial condition to both the lenders and the family, and demonstrating the intent to change one's ways, is a better way out of the fix.

Emerging Trends in Financial Behaviour

There has been a paradigm shift in the way money is pursued, spent and invested, the emphasis being on a 'branded' life and a media-driven aspirational lifestyle—eating out, pubbing, partying, and uninhibitedly spending on personal grooming, pets and travel.

Life is an adventure for which the young are prepared to work extra hard, often in hip workplaces culturally different from traditional work spaces. Long hours of work skew the work–life balance. In addition, there is the social pressure to accomplish milestones early—buying a house, a swanky car and the latest gadgets. The present-day generation is driven. They have internalized the fact that today's global icons[32] include rich businessmen who can fly to the moon on a whim.[33] However, this is an endless quest, as the

---

[32] 'Global Icons', *World Talent Organization*, https://tinyurl.com/4dd9p2ny. Accessed on 13 March 2024.
[33] 'Blue Origin Safely Launches Four Commercial Astronauts to Space and Back', *Blue Origin*, 20 July 2021, https://tinyurl.com/r3jrefzd. Accessed on 13 March 2024.

thrill of a new acquisition or accomplishment is short-lived and is replaced by a new goal of earning, achieving and owning more.

A range of fiscal behaviour can be observed in the present-day generation. Some are financially responsible. Concerned about financial stability, they periodically reassess their situation. In general, such individuals have less economic stress. Some, on the other hand, live in the moment. Impulsive and desirous of instant gratification, they are willing to spend unhesitatingly, to the extent of running up a huge debt on their credit cards.

Be it the cautious type or the risk-taker, economic worries catch up with both. Evaluating the pros and cons at every step can be anxiety-inducing for the cautious people, and if their decisions backfire, they are unable to forgive themselves. As for risk-takers, they should perhaps consult experts rather than assuming that the next time would be lucky for them.

In reality, people are becoming members of the '99 Club', a term for those individuals who are financially sound enough to enjoy their life but are always discontented, longing for that figure of one to complete the metaphorical century. As earning more becomes the prime focus, relationships, health and personal rejuvenation take a back seat. Workaholics don't have a pause button to think about what they are losing in their constant quest to achieve target after target. It would be prudent to set a financial target that is ample for a stress-free life, and to not keep on resetting it.

Consequences of the Money Race

Individuals whose primary goal is to gain the maximum in the shortest time possible never think about what is lost in the process. Money takes precedence over relationships. The innocence and capacity to love and trust starts waning. What remains is only a custodian of wealth.

The stress is unimaginable when a person is in a race with others on the material scale. Initially, it may not feel that the work–life balance is skewed or that it is affecting close relationships, but eventually the effect becomes visible, especially in difficult times when one requires emotional support. One feels a sense of disbelief that one's closest people have become emotionally distant, when in reality, it is just that over time, their complaints have been replaced with detachment and indifference.

A phenomenon known as 'time famine' has come to the fore, referring to the pervasive feeling of shortage of time one has because of being overwhelmed by the demands of work and life.[34] When faced with time famine, money can be seen as both a cause and a potential solution. Monetary affluence often comes with time famine and gives rise to the feeling of 'future time slack' (the belief that one will have more time for oneself in the future if one earns more money today). At the same time, it is a fact that having money also brings with it the luxury of time in the present. The category you belong to out of the two—experiencing time famine or luxury of time—would depend on where you are financially as well

---

[34]Perlow, Leslie A., 'The Time Famine: Toward a Sociology of Work Time', *Administrative Science Quarterly*, Vol. 44, No. 1, 1999, pp. 57–81, https://tinyurl.com/57nvh49d. Accessed on 12 March 2024.

as your priorities and attitude towards life. Essentially, the scarcity of both time and money increases their importance and one's attachment towards them.[35] People reporting time scarcity are less happy and more prone to anxiety, depression, obesity and relationship problems.[36]

Striking a balance is not easy in current times, but it is necessary to try and keep every sphere of life in sync. Moreover, one needs a healthy body and close people around to be able to enjoy the perks of money. Those who like to make investments should invest in their health and relationships just as they do in finance.

It's not just a few individuals wanting an aspirational lifestyle—this longing is the dominant narrative of our society today, as is the myth of striking it rich in one blow. Money, profit and greed are what the world runs on. When desires outstrip ability, there is a tendency to go for questionable shortcuts or even crimes such as digital fraud, money scams and honey-trapping for blackmail, made easy by gadgets. Even one's relatives are not spared. Some even take recourse to gambling and become addicts. These things are true of every segment of our society at this juncture.

By the time reality dawns, it may be too late. Just remember, there is no such thing as a free lunch in today's world. It is up to you to protect yourself from the fantasies spun by some smart advertisement copywriter. The best way

---

[35]Whillans, Ashley, 'Time for Happiness: Why the Pursuit for Money Isn't Bringing You Joy—and What Will', *Harvard Business Review*, 24 January 2019, https://tinyurl.com/bjtjatwb. Accessed on 12 March 2024.

[36]Whillans, Ashley, and Elizabeth Dunn, 'To Promote Happiness, Choose Time Over Money', *Behavioral Scientist*, 14 November 2017, https://tinyurl.com/4x353dyb. Accessed on 12 March 2024.

out: accept the reality of your financial status and work hard to better it, keeping your priorities in sight.

The Way Out

One needs to reflect on money's relationship with happiness. There is no simple solution for a stress-free life in the present-day scenario, where money dominates the imagination. It has been observed that an individual's emotional well-being is definitely directly proportional to money, but only to a certain level. Beyond that, it has the potential to become counterproductive for many.[37] The hard work required to realize one's desires may not leave enough time to savour them.

Thus, it would be wise to choose the lifestyle that goes with your basic worldview. Think hard about how far you want to go to pursue money once your basic comforts are in place, and if you do want to pursue money, whether it is worth all the sacrifice.

It's not easy to differentiate between need and inclination. Ultimately, you need to decide how much is good enough, and whether you should be prudent from the beginning or reassess your work–life balance after achieving a certain milestone. Often people tend to become prisoners of their achievements, and the fear of losing out keeps them going.

If observed minutely, the consequences of pursuing money to the exclusion of everything else are quite visible: friendships start dwindling, and an emotional distance develops in close relationships, with the primary concerns

---

[37]Berger, Michele W., 'Does More Money Correlate with Greater Happiness?', *Penn Today*, 6 March 2023, https://tinyurl.com/4ahr3ze9. Accessed on 12 March 2024.

being purely financial. Health may show signs of early deterioration. Life becomes monotonous, and one eventually reaches the stage of burnout, a state of mental and physical fatigue where one wishes to halt but is bound to carry on. Numbness prevails. Everything may seem fine, but only outwardly. This is the critical point at which you need to evaluate where your life is heading.

Certainly, a better-paying job is a priority, but priorities may and do change with time and financial security. If possible, try doing a job that is meaningful to you, something you *wish* to do rather than are *forced* to do for the money. Also, regularly spending quality time with family, friends and the self and focussing on your health should be an in-built attitude, a way of life that keeps you anchored. It is equally important to enjoy the fruits of your accumulated wealth with people close to you. Plan regular breaks and vacations. Valuing time and relationships is the bedrock of a meaningful life in any and every circumstance.

It goes without saying that reckless spending needs to be checked from the beginning (especially in our economically volatile times), as changing old habits during hardships is not only difficult but traumatic. This is where budgeting helps, by giving insights into actual needs, investments and where one is headed and at what cost. It is important to have plans in place for major expenses like the children's education and one's health. While using credit cards, it is always better to have a realistic rather than presumptuous view of funds and income.

It is quite simple, really. Money helps in fulfilling the inherent human need for comfort and security, but it only helps us to be happy if we know what can and cannot be expected from it.

15

The Price of Prosperity

If there's one word that most people are willing to learn in every living language in today's world, it's the word 'success'. They see the dazzle of economic success, not the reality behind it, namely, that an upward swing in financial worth is as challenging as being in the financial doldrums. Nothing succeeds like success, but the price it extracts in terms of time, energy and effort is considerable.

Generally, the upward climb is slow and steady. Sometimes, fortunes turn suddenly, like when someone gets an extraordinary salary package, makes a killing in the stock market or a land deal, or simply marries into a wealthy family. Accepting this new reality takes time, and the readjustments needed in various spheres of life are a potential stress trigger.

Sudden and intense changes impact the mental framework more. Those from a poor financial background find it more difficult to handle their new affluent circumstances, and they panic early. The age at which economic betterment occurs is also important, as people on the extremes of the age spectrum have less resilience.

The stress generated also depends on the magnitude of

desire for and personal importance given to materialistic success. It helps if one is financially literate. Having an equable personality and supportive family and friends are a help when managing the change.

Managing Wealth

A monetary upswing is a positive development, but the worry about managing it responsibly, the fear of losing it, or the anxiety about the next height to scale can be tremendous.

Managing wealth, figuring out the best way to multiply it, and keeping it safe are more tedious than earning it. Impulsive investments are a no-no. Consulting financial experts is one way to overcome the limitations of inadequate knowledge, indecisiveness and fear of loss. However, wealth generally makes one distrustful of others, which creates anxiety. Enquire about an expert's work from various trusted sources; be transparent and communicative about your financial expectations. Timely and adequate monetary compensation for the expert's services will strengthen the professional relationship and benefit everyone. Keep in mind that sometimes the advice is favourable, and sometimes it is not. In the latter case, avoid playing the blame game and treat it as a learning experience.

Paying more taxes may seem painful to those with new wealth, but it saves you the trouble of making stressful arrangements to remain invisible to the authorities. Honesty brings peace of mind and comfort.

Taking loans to fund one's growth can create anxiety, at least till the desired outcome is realized, and a loss forces many to take extreme steps. Alert decision-making based on weighing the long-term consequences of one's actions is necessary, keeping in mind one's expenditure, investments, savings and standard of living, and various life events and risks.

Despite the stress, the hunger for more keeps one going. Regular introspection on the path being taken, coupled with rejuvenating activities, is needed to ward off mental and physical fatigue. Avoid the stress of comparing yourself with or competing against others. Opting for digital payments can also help ease pressure to a great extent.

Attitudinal Changes

According to well-known American psychologist Abraham Maslow's theory of the hierarchy of needs, once the basic needs (food, clothing, shelter, love and friendship) are secured, the individual yearns for esteem and self-actualization.[38] Some look to social work, philanthropy or politics to build their self-esteem, while for the majority, wealth is associated with power, importance and rewards, and synonymous with societal acknowledgement and high self-esteem.

Money attracts many hangers-on and creates the illusion of the wealthy person being a leader who has all the answers, to the extent that others may be treated as lesser mortals. This impression becomes a belief when even the misplaced opinions of the concerned individual are lauded

---

[38] Maslow, Abraham H., 'A Theory of Human Motivation', *Psychological Review*, Vol. 50, No. 4, 1943, pp. 370–96, https://tinyurl.com/bdh3h545. Accessed on 12 March 2024.

by sycophants. When their views are contested, it leads to egoistic arguments and often spoils relations within the family and even at work.

When that egoistic attitude—'I know everything about everything'—spills over in interactions with experts in other fields, such as doctors and accountants, it creates more problems than solutions. Remaining rooted and treating others as individuals worthy of respect is important.

Many people think that money provides them impunity to flout the law, but that is an erroneous notion and only creates ground for more worries. If it is the adrenaline rush you crave, there is always adventure sport.

Lifestyle Changes

Generally, an upswing in financial status is associated with lifestyle changes tending towards the luxurious—the 'lifestyle creep', as it is called. Easy spending is especially true of those who come into money or inherit wealth.

Some may lead a lifestyle of constantly sporting top brands, which is excessive even for their pockets, telling themselves 'I deserve it, I am worth it', thus often falling into the credit-card debt trap. Each expensive episode leads to confrontations within the family, because it is an unsustainable situation. Growing frustration, detachment and all-round stress can cause irreversible rifts within the family.

If things have gone sideways, it would be sensible to communicate openly with the family and collectively decide what is acceptable and what is not. This goes for everybody, adults as well as children. Containing the damage at the earliest is the first step towards stress resolution. Part of it is inculcating financial discipline, distinguishing between levels of need and luxury, and working within a budget.

Setting boundaries also includes a clear discussion with children about the company they keep and any temptation to explore 'recreational' choices like alcohol or drugs to be part of the smart set, which, apart from being an expensive habit, eventually becomes an addiction. What goes for children goes for adults as well—during times of stress, an escapist urge leads to more trouble, financially, socially and health-wise.

When people rise up the financial ladder, there is a tendency to ape a so-called 'modern' lifestyle, even though there may be some discomfort with it. This includes socializing with members of the opposite sex, which can often take unanticipated turns, lead to extramarital relationships and create an ugly situation within the family. As people leave the security of their rooted, familiar reality, they become vulnerable, and so do their families. Instances of honey-trapping and blackmailing are frequent, what with the ubiquitous smartphone recording intimate moments. The question for such people is: are you willing to lose the confidence of your family for a fleeting guilty pleasure, suffering unimaginable stress as a consequence?

Any activity that involves behaving in a fashion contrary to one's nature puts pressure on a person. Better to pull oneself back in time and change the negative habits triggered by a positive financial condition. Success, as much as failure, shows your character. So, introspect, clear the air with the family, and try to ease the causes of stress so that both your familial relationships and professional situation are solid. For this, it is important to know the exact role that money plays in one's life.

Work-Life Balance

Attaining a superior financial status, and maintaining and improving on it involves consistent hard work, which often messes up one's work–life balance. To many, it boils down to a choice between having less money or less time for the family and self.

From the lives of people around us and those we read about, there is enough information about the cost of success. If you want to stay the course, be clear-headed about charting your life: delegate responsibilities, avoid an emphasis on perfection, create time for family, friends and yourself, and pay heed to your physical and mental health.

Children and Parenting

A higher financial status has a direct impact on children in the sense that the outlook of parents changes. Over-concern, pampering and compensating for lack of time by showering children with gifts are common traits. The entire focus shifts to comforts, not to strengthening the child's capacity to face challenges. When children see every big and little demand fulfilled, they subconsciously start thinking that they are always right, which must be why their demands are being met. Their instinct for struggle reduces to that extent.

Problems arise when children leave the security of home and find it difficult to form relationships or face the outside world's challenges. Unable to confront reality, many fall prey to depression, anxiety and drugs. For parents, it is pure agony to see their child in such a state, which is why they need to observe a sense of proportion in the way they bring up their children right from the start.

Those who have worked to earn money expect their children to share the household's responsibilities once they become older and independent. But pampered children have not been prepared for that—they wonder why they should exert themselves when they have so much. Hence, they turn rebellious, take work casually and make mistakes, or spurn work altogether. This disheartens everyone.

This break in the pattern, going from being pampered to being expected to take on responsibility, can cause depression among children and create conflict in the family. Parents start talking about their own upbringing, but that is of no help.

Parents should know that the foundation of a child's lifelong behaviour is laid early, in the formative years. According to my clinical experience, to ensure that the child has a healthy upbringing, parents can balance rights with responsibilities and rewards with punishments; avoid exposing their children to excess money and comforts, especially at a very young age; not fulfil each and every wish the instant it is conveyed; and promote independence by exposing children to real-life situations, initially under parental guidance and later unassisted.

The first rule of good parenting is that you can't tell children to do something you don't do yourself. Spending responsibly, following a budget and balancing rights and responsibilities with regard to other family members, such as the elders, is bound to set a good example for children.

Moreover, children of successful parents live under their shadow and can wilt under the pressure of expectations to excel in every field. Constant comparison with other children, too, is very stressful as it prevents them from forming friendships with their peers. In such a situation, the parent-child relationship might get stunted. The child may learn only a little about forging strong relationships. When the parents are old, they want their child to look after them. But the child might have little attachment to them, or worse, might see it as an opportunity to teach them a lesson.

Parents should understand that realizing their dreams through their offspring is harmful to the child's development. What they should do, for the best interests of both themselves and the children, is to get to know their children better, appreciate their skills and encourage them to do their best.

Many parents who find it difficult to get through to their troubled youngsters are embarrassed to seek help. They feel they would be judged harshly as people who conquered many frontiers but were unable to keep their home front secure. Realizing the error of one's ways—that the intent was not faulty but the approach was—is the first step towards rectification. Spending time with children and listening to them without being judgemental is the way to start. One may seek the help of a mental health professional if one wants. Things will get better.

Relatives and Others

If learning how to parent in the time of affluence is important, so is learning how to deal with requests of financial help from relatives and friends. It's not an easy situation.

When a loan is not returned on time, it makes the lender restless, leading to repeated reminders, thus jeopardizing the relationship. It is worse when the lender is in need of money but is unable to ask for it as the relationship is delicate. The borrower, who may have valid reasons for nonpayment, feels pressure, guilt and shame with each reminder, which takes a further toll on the relationship.

To keep one's money and relationships secure is a delicate task. The decision to gift or loan money should be taken after considering aspects like the closeness and importance of the relationship, the amount loaned, and the impact if not returned on time or at all. Being transparent about the terms and conditions of a loan is best for everyone concerned. Documentation may seem rude but can help. Otherwise, one may give the money without any expectation of seeing it again, and treat its return as a bonus. To deny the request, though, one shouldn't say no straightaway. Make a plausible excuse. The potential borrower may feel bad initially but will later understand that asking for a loan from you is a no-go.

Here is one precept for anyone who has experienced a financial improvement in life—know the nature of money, what it can do and what it can't. That way, one can enjoy the positives of a comfortable financial situation in one's life.

16

When the Going Tough

Prolonged financial crises or an abrupt setback causing an economic slide can be very stressful. If the change in circumstances occurs over a period—say, due to a divorce, paying back children's education loans, looking after a loved one through illness, making poor financial decisions, or an economic recession—there is some time to adjust, though the pressure never goes away.

A sudden financial setback, particularly after an improvement in one's economic standing, comes as a shock, be it the unexpected demise of a family's sole breadwinner, loss of savings in a Ponzi scheme, or, more commonly, the loss of one's job. This happened in the wake of the Covid-19 pandemic, which forced thousands of businesses to shut down, leaving many people who had made something of their lives jobless and helpless.

Similarly, one can imagine the distress caused by the huge periodic lay-offs in the new economy—the IT sector, global social media companies and e-commerce platforms—which has provided multiple opportunities to the current generation. A job loss can turn people's lives upside down and affect their social, psychological and physical health.

The lifestyle adjustment demanded by a major fall in financial status is painful. There is the fear of being mocked by one's relatives and associates, anger and shame, and the constant thought, 'What could have been done to prevent the financial collapse? Would it be possible to restore one's fortunes?' Unable to face the situation, many, sometimes their families as well, take their own lives, as media reports indicate.

Although difficult, the solution starts with acknowledging reality and then moving on to recovery. Some prefer the escapism of alcohol or drugs, some keep borrowing money to hold on to their earlier lifestyle, and some try to run cons, thus compounding their problems.

The family as a unit should decide how to move ahead. Keep your feet planted on the ground. List your assets and liabilities; explore additional income sources. Selling off assets to pay debts will take some weight off the mind. Financial literacy for better money management is vital for survival.

Job Loss

Our jobs are much more than just a way of making a living. To most of us, they are a valuable part of our identity—how we see ourselves and the way the world perceives us. Jobs also provide structure, purpose and meaning to our lives. The loss of one's job impacts every aspect of life, be it finances, relationships, health or self-esteem. The stress is immense, especially for those in senior positions, for they know that finding similar jobs at their level could be difficult. When there is large-scale unemployment, the impact on society is enormous, as the world witnessed during the course of Covid-19.

Reasons for Job Loss

In recent times, there have been involuntary job losses on a large scale due to automation in some industries and larger circumstances like recession, which trigger cost-cutting measures like retrenchment and outsourcing. As per data, more than 150,000 individuals were laid off globally in the tech sector in 2022. Recent data has also revealed that tech companies worldwide, including those in India, laid off over 1,600 employees per day in 2023.[39]

There are always early indications of such troubles. Sensing and acting on them is being far-sighted. Updating and diversifying skills for a safer job profile in the same firm or elsewhere, and focussing on increasing financial savings will stave off anxiety to a considerable extent. To think that nothing can happen to you is pseudo-optimism.

Companies find it cheaper to hire newcomers than to retain current workers who have to be paid more. One needs to constantly upgrade one's skills to remain in business, providing the promise of something extra that experience and knowledge bring, which is essential for a company's fortunes.

If you are someone who prefers to work within a structure, realize that every organization has its own work culture and you must be aware of it. You should be able to read your senior's indirect comments on your work and behaviour. Reflect on them or sound out trusted colleagues and do what is required to clear the air—the sooner the better.

---

[39]'Recession Fears: Tech Companies Laying off 1,600 Workers per Day in 2023, and It's Increasing', *The Economic Times*, 17 January 2023, https://tinyurl.com/4w53z4hb. Accessed on 13 March 2024.

Sometimes, a poorly defined job description or a senior's toxic behaviour may create a precarious situation. Tackling it head-on, 'for I am right', may help you in the short term, but it can lead to a protracted ego clash, damaging your long-term prospects. An assertive attitude involving a one-to-one talk with the employer to define your role and the expectations from it would be more fruitful. Remember, sometimes performance alone may not be able to save you, so be pragmatic and bide your time till the next job comes along.

There are other reasons for job loss—for example one's reluctance to relocate, or family circumstances like having to look after a parent in illness. Such decisions are difficult and should be made only after considering the short- and long-term consequences of opting out of that job and remaining unemployed. Only then should one plan one's next move.

In other scenarios, some people may decide to put in their papers after experiencing burnout or getting tired of an unfulfilling job. Some may leave with plans for a start-up in mind. Plan carefully and make sure there are enough funds to fall back on. Opt for a sabbatical (if that's an option) or unpaid leave rather than resigning. Keep Plan B handy in case your original plan does not match expectations.

Impacts of Job Loss

Whatever the reason for the loss of a job may be, it is always traumatic as somewhere along the way your job becomes your dominant identity. For someone who relishes the challenges and compensations of a job, it can be doubly distressing.

The level of stress created by the loss of one's job depends on one's financial stability, age, chances of re-employment, family and social support, interpersonal relations at work, work experience, and whether one has been adequately compensated for one's loyalty. If fired, stress levels depend also on how one has been removed—unceremoniously or respectfully. Whatever the reason, coping with joblessness isn't easy.

Emotions after Job Loss

Any transition in one's work life is taxing, let alone job loss. Some may turn towards self-contemplation, but most people experience psychological hardships. There is a sense of disbelief but most of all, there is also a loss of professional identity, power and purpose in life. The loss of self-esteem and social confidence is accompanied by frustration, resentment, self-pity, humiliation and apprehension about the future. Such situations can trigger anxiety and depression, and lead to self-harming behaviour.

Grief and negativity are understandable, but the sooner one initiates corrective efforts, the better. Try to accept reality at the earliest. Remember, your job is an important part of your identity, but it is not the only parameter for defining who you are in totality.

Moreover, self-blame will give rise to sadness and affect your chances of future employment. Give yourself time to adjust. See the situation as an opportunity to reconsider priorities, overcome deficiencies, and develop resilience. Rather than brood over the unfairness of it, it's better to ventilate your feelings in front of those you trust. Avoid judgemental and negative people while sharing your emotions.

Behaviour after Job Loss

The loss of a job impacts not just the person but their entire family as well. A high-strung person is likely to be impacted more. There is a marked tendency to shun society, withdraw into one's shell and brood. Remember, mental stress will affect your future job prospects and your relationships. Make an attempt to be with positive people—emotions are contagious, after all. Even if one prides oneself on being strong and self-sufficient, one should not hesitate to take the support offered by people who care. Relationships are not just about sharing happy moments; they are about caring for each other in stressful times as well.

Many people turn to alcohol or drugs as a way to cope with stress and to kill time. A temporary escape, it only negatively impacts finances, relationships, health and re-employment possibilities.

It is more important to maintain a daily routine that includes focussing on self-care. One can adopt a health regimen (including exercise, yoga, meditation, proper sleep and a balanced diet). Daily acts of kindness act as stress busters and are a diversion from one's own problems. Moreover, one should take the time to re-evaluate one's life and upgrade one's skills. Be in shape for the next job; opportunity knocks at the door of those who are prepared for it. That's what being 'future ready' means.

If you are unable to control the intensity of your emotions and behaviour, do not have reservations about taking professional help. It is not a sign of weakness. Moreover, professionals may help you see the situation in a new light.

Impact on the Domestic Front

It is necessary to do everything it takes to steady oneself as joblessness puts great pressure on familial relationships. Facing the heat of the downward slide, family members may hold the individual responsible for the job loss and vocalize their displeasure both publicly and privately.

The family is one's first support system. It should be non-judgemental, supportive and motivating. See that arguments don't turn into ego hassles, causing permanent damage.

Financial Impact

The loss of a job means drying up of a regular source of income (and savings). Its impact depends on the level of savings and expenditure, whether there's another source of income and if the person will be able to handle any unexpected expense. Finally, the person's attitude towards money—whether one is a spendthrift, miser or judicious spender—is important. A person who has been careful about saving money, making investments, and having insurance and medical policies from day one of working would be better placed. Returns from investments can act as a source of income when faced with job loss.

Still, apprehensions abound regarding one's ability to get another job, and how a serious financial crunch may affect one's ability to look after the family. Men who are still attuned to the traditional social expectation of being the primary providers feel more inadequate, even if their spouses are working.

Don't look away. To get a grip on life and to know exactly where you stand, start writing your current income and expenses in detail. That will enable you to weed out expenses that are not basic. Simplifying life—through steps like shifting to a smaller residence, replacing your big car with a smaller one, eating at home, using a less expensive cell phone—can ease your stress. If re-employment seems a distant prospect, do what it takes to reduce EMIs, which may even mean selling off some assets. If needed, consult trusted friends or experts. After all, mental health is more important than maintaining a certain lifestyle.

Finding a New Job

Whether you resign due to unpleasant circumstances or for a better paying job, or are fired, never leave on a bad note, no matter how upset you feel. You may need references. Moreover, friendly ex-colleagues may provide a lead for another job.

The truth is that the vast majority of jobs are never advertised. Truly, your network is your net worth. Don't hesitate to tap into this network. Everyone is aware of uncertain job scenarios, and you are not the lone victim. The more people there are who know what you want, the more help you get in being introduced to prospective employers.

Don't delay creating a job-search plan with defined goals and manageable steps. Be patient and focus on things that are in your control, such as upgrading your skills, contacting headhunters, exploring Internet job portals, and setting up meetings (physical or virtual) with your contacts.

One's age, the period of unemployment, and the financial and market conditions play a role in the kind of job one may get. The new job could pay less, be seen as a demotion, or require travel or relocation. Some will accept this for they are clear they want a fixed monthly income. Others may think it is beneath them. However, reality and need should have the upper hand over pride. It is better to work than stay idle. Once back in circulation, the chances of being noticed and getting a better job are higher.

Losing a job can be harrowing, but it is not the end of the world. Recasting your future will be easier if you are at your best—mentally, emotionally and physically. So, accept reality, count your blessings, and move on to the next phase of life. As a purposeful human being, that should be your primary job.

17

The Lows of a High

There was a time when there was greater stigma attached to individuals struggling with substance use. A person 'on drugs' was seen as morally deficient. Today, there is greater awareness that substance use disorder is a mental health problem and needs to be treated as such.

The term 'substance' here refers to a psychoactive substance, one that targets the psyche. The term is used interchangeably with alcohol and/or other drugs. 'Substance use disorder' is a term covering the entire spectrum of consumption, encompassing abuse, harmful use and dependence/addiction.

These terms are overlapping. Abuse refers to persistent and injudicious use. Harmful use is said to happen when substance use causes actual physical or mental damage (e.g., liver illness, depression). It can happen even with a single episode or over a few episodes of substance consumption; e.g., sharing a needle for intravenous drug use can lead to hepatitis, or an accident can happen during one's first use of alcohol. Dependence or addiction is a cluster of physiological, behavioural and cognitive phenomena, where the use of a substance is characterized by an intense desire for it, difficulty in controlling substance-taking behaviour, withdrawal symptoms on stopping or decreasing the quantity of substance, development of tolerance to its effects, neglect of alternative pleasures or interests, and persisting with substance use despite clear evidence of harmful consequences. This substance use pattern leads to significant impairments in health and social and occupational functioning. Addiction takes time to build.[40]

Psychoactive substances alter neurochemicals, making a person feel euphoric, energetic, mentally alert and talkative, and are repeatedly, compulsively consumed to experience the same pleasurable effects. Even if one knows that they cause socio-occupational damage, they become one's only priority in life and the only way to achieve pleasure. Moreover, one requires an increasing quantity to experience the same amount of pleasure. Attempts to decrease or stop the intake produce withdrawal symptoms. This is known as addiction.

Alcohol and nicotine (tobacco, cigarettes, etc.) are the most common substances of abuse that are legal and easily available, with the former accepted as an integral part of socializing. However, there are laws governing their sale and promotion.

The consumption of legal and illegal substances (cannabis, opioids, cocaine and hallucinogens) is increasing across sections of our society. Moreover, the average age of users has been decreasing steadily to include even school-going children. The chances of addiction increase

---

[40]World Health Organization, *The ICD-10 Classification of Mental and Behavioural Disorders: Clinical Descriptions and Diagnostic Guidelines*, 1992, https://tinyurl.com/3e6t24pp. Accessed on 12 March 2024.

when unhealthy substance use starts at a young age.

Indian law on legal and illegal substance use is stringent. Yet, their easy availability, from right outside schools to the poshest of places, is cause for worry. The trade in illegal substances thrives on inelastic demand, which constantly increases the catchment of vulnerable individuals.

Identifying the reasons for the increasing incidence of harmful substance use is important for prevention. People often say that it helps them overcome stress, deal with difficult emotions like frustration and anger, and feel relaxed. It begins to seem like the only way to function better, leading to addiction over time.

Peer pressure is also a major reason, especially for youngsters, as is a sense of adventure. For some, substance use is a status symbol and a sign of independence. An independent existence in cities as well as easy availability and affordability are contributing factors. Neglect or addiction in the family, and a genetic predisposition to addiction, also have a role to play.

Learning and practising positive ways to tackle stress and its causes are preventive factors. Being assertive and saying no to peers, airing one's feelings and discussing problems with trusted family members and friends are effective ways to handle stress, as are introspection and working on available solutions. Developing a physical regimen is also desirable. Many high achievers fool themselves by insisting that they are not addicted. They, too, need to introspect and consult professionals if needed.

Overcoming peer pressure is important. True friends will never force you into a difficult situation. Think hard—will your 'friends' accept their role in pushing you towards substance dependence and be willing to share the treatment cost? If the answer is no, then they are not your friends.

Adolescence: A Crucial Time

During adolescence, youngsters seek independence, become rebellious, and look for new experiences without recognizing the consequences of their actions. Negative home environment, poor academic performance, difficulty with interpersonal skills, a history of physical or sexual abuse, underdeveloped coping mechanisms, peer pressure, harmful use of substances by a parent, and easy availability of psychoactive substances propel adolescents towards them.

Harmful substance use during teenage years affects an individual's mental and emotional growth, and may give rise to violent and age-inappropriate sexual behaviour, minor and major crimes, and higher chances of mental disorders or suicidal urges.[41] Academics and relationships are also negatively impacted. Most adolescents deny that they are taking substances and resist treatment. Observing a decline in their academics, relationships and health, the parents focus their energies on them. This may also lead to siblings feeling ignored.

Hence, it is important for parents to be attuned to their children's lives—not to be controlling but to be connected to

---

[41] Office of Juvenile Justice and Delinquency Prevention, *Drug Identification and Testing in the Juvenile Justice System*, May 1998, pp. 4–9, https://tinyurl.com/3xypt3h3. Accessed on 13 March 2024; Nebhinani, Naresh, Pranshu Singh, and Mamta, 'Substance Use Disorders in Children and Adolescents', *Journal of Indian Association for Child and Adolescent Mental Health*, Vol. 18, No. 2, 2022, pp. 128–36, https://tinyurl.com/3urs7mpv. Accessed on 13 March 2024.

them, especially in a nuclear family. Communication is vital—parents need to listen without being judgemental. A mix of firmness and openness helps the child confide in parents. Instead of goading them into pursuing more achievements, parents should inspire the youngsters to imbibe coping skills and patience and value emotional balance by practising these themselves.

It's important to catch the telltale signs: being withdrawn and secretive; now excitable, now drowsy, now rebellious. Red eyes, nicotine marks on fingers, a new set of friends, increased demands for money, a tendency to steal money, and falling academic grades tell a story. Upon searching, discovery of suspicious substances in wallets, bags or drawers is an important indicator. Urine and breath analyser tests are the surest way to ascertain harmful substance use in the face of denial. Upon confirmation, parents should make sure to broach the subject in a gentle and compassionate manner.

Placing too many restrictions on teenagers makes them want to experiment. It is better to educate them about acceptable and unacceptable use, and recreational and irresponsible use. Parents need to be good role models. If a parent realizes that they too have a problem with recognizing their own limits, they should accept it and make an effort to resolve it.

Adolescents should be counselled that rights and responsibilities always coexist. With their right to seek emotional and financial support from the family comes the responsibility to maintain a healthy lifestyle and concentrate on their personal growth.

Parents should also tell the adolescent that between the Internet and the doctor, it's the latter's word that is final.

After all, international health agencies do recognize the abuse and dependence potential of these substances.

Negotiate to provide real and acceptable alternative choices, from exercise to hobbies and interests. Along with medical treatment, parents should be open to individual or family counselling. Encouragement of agreeable behaviour helps the child's confidence.

Rehabilitation after a detox is a painfully long process. Without making it apparent, it would be prudent to keep an eye on the youngster, acting at the slightest hint rather than waiting for the problem to become bigger.

For long-term rehabilitation, the adolescent should be encouraged to develop an alternate, non-harmful support system comprising family members, teetotaller friends and good coping mechanisms. Keeping them busy with various pursuits helps. A family member may have to accompany the youngster during the initial period.

◆

With older people, the harmful use of prescription drugs and alcohol is likelier. Distress due to physical, psychological, financial or emotional ill-treatment pushes them towards drugs, especially painkillers and sedatives.

Weaning them off or putting them on alternate medicines to control the underlying illness is not easy. Counselling, too, may have a limited influence at that age. Active family support plays a major role. Being available and listening to them is important—support should be given in actions, not only in words. For geriatric persons, any weaning off should be done under the doctor's guidance.

The Social Impact of Harmful Substance Use

Substance dependence has far-reaching and complex social impacts depending on the family structure, age and gender of the person, responsibilities, financial and social support, and any other existing condition, such as a mental disorder. The closest family members suffer the most.

The most common scenario is the man in the family having an addiction problem, leading to him becoming emotionally almost cut-off from the family and not fulfilling his responsibilities. The household suffers intense negativity, altercations and mental trauma. Domestic violence creates an environment of hate and fear; sometimes legal protection is sought. Misdirected anger, guilt and self-medication are common coping strategies. Afraid of losing face, some families may live in denial.

If there are financial burdens, the family's displeasure towards the person suffering addiction increases. Generally, the partner is the worst affected, having to play the role of both parents in raising the children while facing loneliness and complete detachment. Frustrated, the partner may seek solace outside the marriage, with separation or divorce on the cards.

As for the children, every aspect of their lives—childhood, education, health, personality development and emotional stability—is affected. More likely to face abuse (physical and sexual) and neglect, they live in denial and fear. Parental inconsistency in setting rules and enforcing them leads to erratic behaviour. Feeling responsible for their parent's substance problem, they may assume adult responsibilities early. They may also show a greater propensity for harmful substance use, violence, mental disorders, and adjustment and relationship problems. Conversely, their intense hatred for substances may make them controlling and overprotective parents later on. The effects continue for generations.

It is important that the family accepts the reality before they do. Figuring out whether the domestic problems preceded or followed harmful substance use is futile. Both mutually reinforce each other, hence family therapy and addiction treatment need to be simultaneous.

Remember, addiction is a brain disorder. Help is needed for de-addiction. Detoxification and rehabilitation both require medication and counselling. Along with medicines, willpower helps in abstention. Calling and talking to a professional is always the first step.

Health Impacts (Physical, Mental and Sexual Health)

In terms of physical health, addiction leaves no organ untouched, be it brain, heart, lungs, liver, kidney or gastrointestinal system. It also affects hormonal and reproductive systems. Long-term use is associated with cancer, and proneness to sexually transmitted diseases and infections. Moreover, substances and mental disorders have a reciprocal relationship. Depression, aggression, psychosis and antisocial personality disorder commonly coexist alongside harmful substance use, so do impaired cognition, loneliness and suicidal thoughts. As for their impact on sexual health, initially substances may enhance desire and performance, but these usually go downhill in the long term.

For any medical treatment to work, the person has to stop using substances altogether.

Professional, Economic and Legal Impact

Professionally, one faces a loss of productivity and employability. Over time, one may start using substances during work hours as well. Holding a job may become difficult. Colleagues who have to do the heavy lifting are bound to become resentful.

Moreover, consuming substances and dealing with its health impacts cost money. Gambling, a common habit among those struggling with addiction, often adds to the financial burden. Court battles over property disputes, loan defaults, divorce and child custody rights are also common. Crime (both minor and major) frequently becomes a companion, which may result in a prison term.

The Way Out

Ideally, prevention is the best solution to addiction, but for those who are struggling with it, the success of treatment depends on the person's age, financial condition and level of motivation, the duration of harmful use and its health impacts, and the extent of familial support.

It is vital to overcome the erroneous and dangerous belief that one's dependence is not harmful, and that it is the only way one has of coping with the exceptional circumstances of life. The sooner help is sought, the earlier the turnaround. Treatment can be initiated by the person struggling with addiction or a family member. A clinical assessment is necessary to understand the severity of impact, underlying issues, and motivation to recover from the addiction.

Motivation can and does change with time and stressors, but one must realize that nobody is powerless. Through medicine and counselling, recovery is possible. A supportive family and self-reminders enhance motivation.

Depending on the substance in question, detoxification begins by completely stopping or slowly tapering its consumption. Troublesome withdrawal symptoms are managed by medication. Sometimes, a better option is replacement with non-addictive or less addictive medication, which is then tapered off.

Craving is dealt with in the next phase of rehabilitation, which focusses on understanding and tackling the reasons behind addiction to maintain the state of abstinence. It involves medicines and counselling (individual, family or group therapy). Mental and physical illnesses have to be simultaneously addressed. A person can opt for either inpatient or outpatient detox and rehab.

It is a myth that the medicines used to treat addiction are addictive. As the dosage generally does not change even for long periods, they do not lead to dependence.

Relapses, though avoidable, are very common and expected, and should not lead to discouragement. Exploring the reasons behind them and attempting again is the answer.

Dependence or addiction is a trait of the brain. The brain requires something to depend on, either a substance or a behaviour; it recognizes pleasure, no matter how it gets it. Dependence on or addiction to substances is bad dependence—the pleasure is fleeting, achieved without major physical effort, and is damaging. In the case of good behavioural dependence, it takes major physical/mental effort to achieve pleasure—playing a sport, going to the gym, cooking, gardening, altruism—and it is extremely rewarding in the long run, apart from being socially acceptable. The trick is to discover one's inclination and pursue it wholeheartedly.

It is difficult to answer this question: 'If drugs are so dangerous, why are they so easily available?' The fact is that alcohol and tobacco are legally obtainable but are governed by restrictions. Substances like cannabis and opioids have medicinal use but they are available illegally also. Why and how we use a substance is what makes it useful or harmful.

Substances are not a tool to fight or evade emotions with. Sooner or later, their impact on the body and one's life becomes visible. So why not learn a better coping mechanism to overcome difficult life circumstances?

18

Let's Talk about Sex and Sexuality

For a long time, before film censorship guidelines in India became more liberal, generations of cinema lovers decoded scenes showing two flowers swaying towards each other as a proxy for sexual play between the hero and the heroine.

Similarly, a couple of generations in urban centres have grown up seeing advertisements on walls, tree trunks and behind autorickshaws about people who can set *mardana kamzori* (erectile dysfunction) right, and make life pleasurable.

Both these instances exemplify a certain societal mindset: openness about sexual matters in Indian society, God forbid!

The continuing veil of secrecy on such issues is problematic, for the issue of sexual dysfunction (any issue due to which one or both partners fail to achieve gratification from sexual intercourse) is not uncommon. A companionable sexual relationship is necessary not just for procreation but also for the experience of pleasure that draws partners emotionally closer, especially if they are at the beginning of their journey.

Sexual dysfunction can occur at any stage of the sexual process—from not having any desire for sexual activity (libido) to problems of physical arousal or during orgasm.

Quite often, it is the differing levels of libido among partners that become an issue. According to my clinical experience, the problem of low desire is seen more commonly among women.

During the arousal stage, the problem males could experience is of erectile dysfunction—difficulty in getting an erection or sustaining it for the act to end satisfactorily—whereas women face the problem of not having enough vaginal lubrication.

In the final stage of orgasm, the problem shows up either as early orgasm or premature ejaculation, which fails to gratify either or both partners, or as a delayed orgasm, prolonging the act to an extent that it becomes monotonous, tiring and frustrating. In my professional experience, the problem among women is the inability to achieve orgasm. Moreover, penetrative sex may be painful for some women, resulting in its avoidance. Any of the above, alone or in combination, is cause for dissatisfaction and hence a concern.

Men and women of all ages experience sexual dysfunction, but its prevalence increases with age. Among men, premature ejaculation is the most common sexual complaint. Women are more prone to reporting low sexual desire, pain during sex and delayed/no orgasm.

Sexual dysfunction is linked to a person's emotional, mental and medical state. Stress is the most common trigger (as well as product) of sexual problems, and it could be due to professional or personal issues, or past trauma such as sexual abuse. At times, it is the patriarchal mindset that creates stress—the glorification of male virility often becomes a source of anxiety for young men, whereas women in their marriages are culturally conditioned to fulfil the sexual needs of their partners and not expected to demonstrate a sex drive. Burdened by sexual inhibitions, many women perceive themselves to be sexually inadequate and are thus not motivated enough for sexual activity. The eventual result is low sexual desire and orgasmic dysfunction. In many cases, the oft-repeated myth that sexual intercourse is very painful makes them psychosomatically experience such pain.

However, the scenario is changing, especially in cities. Economically independent women living on their own, with a firmer sense of self, are becoming assertive about their sexual needs as well. Due to changing cultural norms, the taboos associated with premarital sex and virginity are slackening. The present-day generation is more upfront in expressing sexual desire.

The Pressure of the First Time

The root of male sexual dysfunction can often be traced to one's first sexual performance. Lack of experience coupled with a tendency for comparison, fuelled by peers' boasts or explicit sexual videos, leads to performance anxiety. Some may feel rushed, worry that there is a point to be proven or that they may not be able to fulfil the partner's assumed expectations, or feel a fear of being caught out.

Some may have qualms about doing the 'wrong' thing, especially if the people having sex are not married, but still go along with it because they feel saying no would mean the end of the relationship. A word of advice: such issues have more to do with the boundaries people set for themselves regarding what is acceptable for them. One must not feel pressured into giving in if one is not comfortable. Also, it is important to be aware of safe sex practices.

A first-time experience that satisfies both partners creates positivity. But if the man's anxiety results in an inability to achieve or sustain erection and/or culminates in early ejaculation, it can create guilt and even lead to avoidance of sexual activity, which, in turn, increases anxiety. If this experience occurs before marriage, then some individuals may even avoid or delay their marriage on one pretext or another.

Women, too, get impacted if they do not achieve sexual release through orgasm, but many do not express their feelings due to their cultural conditioning, and are often reluctant to discuss the subject.

At a young age, stress due to emotional/psychological reasons largely accounts for sexual dysfunction. Problems may also increase with age due to medical reasons.

Dealing with Stress for Sexual Health

The mantra of *samay*, *suraksha*, *sahyog* (time, safety, cooperation) can help young couples lead a healthy sexual life if followed correctly.[42]

First, the time (adequate time for and adequately timed sexual activity): sex should not be a hurried affair—the couple should have adequate time for arousal through foreplay. Second, sexual activity should be undertaken only

---

[42]Psychiatrist Now, 'सेक्स समस्या का इतना आसान समाधान Sexual Problems? Reasons and Treatments, Solutions Call- 9911887706', *YouTube*, https://tinyurl.com/bdh4hxbw. Accessed on 13 March 2024.

when both partners are feeling energetic and not drained after a long day of work in office or at home. Be flexible and inventive and cooperate with each other to explore a suitable time for it. Switching off digitally also provides time to regenerate sex drive.

Second is safety, both mental and sexual. One should protect oneself by shedding myths and cultural narratives that induce guilt and inadequacy. Partners should educate themselves, talk to each other or to more experienced, trusted friends. While having sex, they must ensure they have privacy so that they feel physically secure to make the process pleasurable. The assurance of sex in privacy relaxes the mind and makes enjoyment possible.

The third aspect is cooperation. When the partners give each other pleasure, they come closer. A one-sided act is often disastrous—the man may wonder if he is being too demanding or whether he has it in him to satisfy his partner, and the woman might wonder what it's all about. Mental blocks should be directly and unhesitatingly discussed with the companion or through a trusted interlocutor. Continuous sexual frustration can result in marital discontent.

Most often, it is the difference in the libido of partners which produces frustration, uncooperative sexual activity and disappointment. It would be wise to meet each other halfway and arrive at a decided frequency of sexual activity. The predictability of the act can make it monotonous, but if partners ask each other about the fantasies that excite them, then it becomes a totally different experience. During the act, erotic aids (in the form of specific clothes, sensual dance, sexually explicit material, etc.) and erotic language, introduced by either or both partners, can help reignite the spark.

If these aspects are considered, the chances of anxiety during sex lessen, and the couple experiences intimate bonding. If the problem persists, then it is better to seek medical help.

The Burden of Sexual Beliefs and Myths

Sexual attitudes, feelings and behaviours are innate or generally developed by observing the behaviour of people around oneself. Circumstances shape many of the sexual beliefs that play a vital role in leading to sexual dysfunction.

Take the widely prevalent myths about masturbation being unhealthy and immoral and that it leads to the wastage of 'sacred' semen. The narrative is that erectile dysfunction is linked to excessive masturbation, commonly referred to as 'childhood mistakes'. Any whitish substance in urine is wrongly considered semen and is associated with causing weakness. There are myriad misconceptions regarding the dimensions of the penis as well.

Sex education from a reliable source at the right age—around puberty—is the answer. It includes knowing one's body and its functions, maintaining hygiene, realizing the connection between physical and emotional intimacy, destroying the damaging myths about sexual habits, and learning about the age of consent and safe sex. There is much to learn about the physiological, psychological and sociological aspects of sexual response and reproduction.

The concept of formal sex education in India is still almost nonexistent. The predominant sources of sex education are friends and media, including the Internet, which are not always dependable. Ideally, parents and teachers are best suited for the task, but they are either too embarrassed to deal with it or think it will increase sexual activity in children. Hence, few youngsters are prepared for the sexual awkwardness or difficulties they encounter due to sheer ignorance.

Therefore, it is always advisable to shed one's inhibitions and seek help from informed individuals (parents, friends, teachers, healthcare providers, etc.). A non-judgemental attitude is essential to connect with youngsters. Ultimately, this education empowers individuals to make informed decisions about their sexuality, and helps prevent sexual abuse and violence.

Common Life Circumstances

Various physiological changes in women's reproductive cycle including the premenstrual syndrome, pregnancy, childbirth and menopause generally decrease their libido, eventually affecting sexual frequency. Even couples who have a vigorous sexual life get impacted. Instead of feeling frustrated and ignored, men need to be supportive of their partners in such circumstances; they can satisfy their own sexual urges through masturbation.

With age, responsibilities increase, and physical stamina decreases. Simultaneously, there are hormonal changes in both sexes and a corresponding decrease in sexual desire and frequency of sexual activity. The initial sympathy and understanding may give way to fights if avoidance continues for long. This may also happen if there are other stress-generating factors such as work-related burdens, poor work–life balance, marital and family disagreements, extramarital affairs, or mental and physical fatigue. Depression and anxiety disorders also impact desire and performance.

Many couples live in denial, saying the problems are situational and will get resolved on their own. Often there is deliberate avoidance on both sides—reaching home late, opting for night shifts, asking the children to sleep alongside them, watching the screen till late, or sleeping (or pretending to sleep) before the partner comes to bed.

These are not solutions. Ideally, partners should be supportive of each other and consultation should be sought, as it is a treatable medical condition.

Seeking Consultation

Even if the incidence of sexual dysfunction is higher in women, it's mostly men who seek help, for they are culturally conditioned to equate the sexual act with manhood, while a low sex drive for women is taken as normal behaviour.

As women are becoming more assertive, the scenario is changing. Not only do they persuade their partners to take proper treatment, they have started approaching doctors for their sexual issues as well. Their problems are generally discovered in the course of examination for mental health issues (depression, anxiety, etc.) or in the aftermath of marital conflict.

Whom to Approach and What the Treatment Entails

Considering the deafening silence on sexual matters in Indian society, it needs to be understood that sexual dysfunction is a medical illness like other illnesses and a doctor holding a proper medical degree should be approached for it.

The medical specialists who can help in these matters are psychiatrists, endocrinologists and urologists. As the individual's disturbed emotional and mental state is the most common reason and consequence of sexual dysfunction, the first point of contact should be a mental health professional.

Decreased sexual desire is a major symptom of depression. Erectile dysfunction and premature ejaculation can cause or result from anxiety disorder, and sometimes, sexual problems improve following treatment of anxiety and depression. In such cases, the treatment depends on the intensity of depression and anxiety: milder illnesses may need lifestyle changes, psychotherapy and some medicines, while moderate to severe illness should be initially addressed through medicines. To regain confidence and sexual potential, medicines to improve erection and delay orgasm may be required.

Simultaneously, there is a need to work on family issues and poor work–life balance. Couples therapy is an option—couples are given periodic assignments that help in rejuvenating their sex life.

Apart from psychological factors, various medical disorders (anatomical, vascular, hormonal, neurological, etc.), poor nutrition, certain medications' side effects and regular intake of alcohol and tobacco can impact sexual function. Treating underlying medical conditions, improving nutrition, replacing medication that has the side effect of hampering sexual activity with other medicines, and discontinuation of intoxicants are the main treatment principles.

It is vital to rule out physical causes of sexual dysfunction by conducting relevant investigations, especially in older age. In the event of any abnormality, consult an endocrinologist for hormonal disturbance, a urologist for anatomical disturbance, and a dermatologist for infections. Quacks masquerading as sexologists should be avoided at all costs.

Beyond all this, understanding each other's viewpoint and accordingly making adjustments to reach common ground is required. Work towards it if that is what you desire. Remember, a healthy sex life keeps you on an even keel in all aspects of life, personal or professional.

Challenges Faced by the LGBTQ+ Community

It is also important to recognize that the challenges are amplified for individuals belonging to the LGBTQ+ community, who often face stigma, discrimination, abuse and exclusion in different spheres of life.

For LGBTQ+ individuals, societal prejudices and marginalization compound their struggles, leaving them vulnerable to exploitation. The youth, in particular, are much more vulnerable since they don't have the guidance and the support system they need at a time when they are coming to terms with their orientation. Some might not even realize their sexual orientation and/or gender identity, and rely on conventional norms as propagated by society. This can lead to dissatisfaction with their life, which can later develop into a cause of stress or anxiety.

Furthermore, being emotionally and financially dependent on their families makes them vulnerable to force, abuse (verbal and physical) and emotional blackmail under the false assumption that their identity can be altered by counselling and conversion therapy. This lack of acceptance by the family and society can lead to serious mental health problems, drug addiction, self-harm tendencies and risky sexual behaviour.

If they are lucky enough to have the family's support and the benefit of a good education, they may land a good job. However, at work they are forced to hide their identity; else they are subjected to discrimination and ridicule. Their capabilities are quite often judged not on the basis of their performance but in light of their sexual/gender identity.

Understanding the concepts of gender and sexuality is essential in addressing these issues sensitively. While unconventional sexual orientations and gender identities are increasingly being recognized as natural variations of the human experience, societal attitudes and language can still perpetuate harmful stereotypes and stigma. Efforts to educate society and promote inclusivity are critical for improving the well-being of LGBTQ+ individuals. There has been progress towards greater acceptance and inclusion, with events like Pride Month helping raise awareness and providing support. However, prejudice and discrimination persist, causing significant stress and emotional turmoil.

Addressing the mental health issues within the LGBTQ+ community requires a multifaceted approach. Healthcare professionals must be trained to provide culturally competent care and support, while families and communities must actively work to create safe and supportive environments. Legal protections against discrimination and hate crimes are also essential steps towards fostering a more inclusive society.

Ultimately, the journey towards destigmatizing and supporting the LGBTQ+ community requires collective effort and ongoing advocacy. LGBTQ+ people suffer not because they are a minority but because the majority is prejudiced. We are all humans; let us not put labels on each other. Labelling can alter life's course and direction.

19

When Virtual Becomes Reality

If people were to keep a daily journal of what they did in today's world, their entries might be annoyingly repetitive: 'Woke up in the morning, checked my phone for messages. Before sleeping at night, checked the phone for messages. Kept the smartphone by my side all day long.'

Globally, more and more people are riding the Internet highway on their smartphones, turning their devices into a one-stop shop for information, entertainment, social media, games and finances. An increasing number seem to prefer the virtual world accessed on the phone screen to the realities of personal, social, student and professional life, and that is a big, big problem.

Like dependence on substances, smartphone dependence, also known as Internet addiction disorder and screen addiction, is becoming a reality of our times. Dependence indicates the level of difficulty in controlling its use despite the harmful consequences.

According to Nielsen's India Internet Report 2023, India had over 700 million Internet users and over 450 million smartphone users as of December 2022.[43] These numbers are bound to rise as there are over 1 billion mobile phone users in the country and given the proliferation of easily accessible and increasingly affordable means to connect to the Internet, user-friendly smartphones and apps. With the introduction of 5G services, the Internet experience is poised to become even better. Hence, there is a need to understand what smartphone dependence and Internet addiction disorder are all about.

Dependence is characterized by:

- preoccupation with the smartphone;
- euphoria generated by accessing the Internet on the smartphone;
- regular upgradation of the device;
- gradually increased duration of use;
- irritability or anxiety caused by efforts to control or stop use;
- retrospective guilt over excessive use;
- sleep deprivation and/or distortion;
- using the smartphone as an escape from real-life problems;
- social withdrawal and fatigue;
- secrecy, need for privacy and creating multiple personas online;
- higher stress levels; and
- negative socio-occupational consequences.

In the course of daily use, the boundary between justified use (need) and dependence gets blurred. A person accessing

---

[43]'India Had over 700 Mn Active Internet Users by Dec '22: Report', *Economic Diplomacy Division, Ministry of External Affairs*, 16 March 2023, https://tinyurl.com/y6f6aknu. Accessed on 13 March 2024.

the Internet all day long as part of the job is *using* it, while one hooked on it for enjoyment or escapism at the expense of one's socio-occupational life is *dependent* on it. During the pandemic, when the world went online to maintain physical isolation, both aspects—use and dependence—increased dramatically.

Over time, the activities of dependence have shifted from emailing, messaging and chatting to social interaction or cyber-relationship addiction, information overload, role-playing games, gambling and pornography. Gaming addiction is most common, followed by addictive Internet browsing and porn addiction. Research shows that neurobiologically these activities on the Internet are similar to dependence on substances.[44]

China was the first country to officially classify Internet addiction as a clinical problem, and started clinics for its treatment.[45] In India, the National Institute of Mental Health and Neurosciences (NIMHANS), Bengaluru, started the Service for Healthy Use of Technology (SHUT) clinic in April 2014 to tackle digital dependence, something that other institutions have since emulated.[46] Now, NIMHANS also has a dedicated helpline number for overcoming tech addiction.

---

[44]Darnai, Gergely, et al., 'Internet Addiction and Functional Brain Networks: Task-Related fMRI Study', *Scientific Reports*, Vol. 9, No. 1, 2019, https://tinyurl.com/33ffrrsc. Accessed on 25 April 2024.

[45]Jiang Qiaolei, 'Development and Effects of Internet Addiction in China', *Oxford Research Encyclopedia of Communication*, 2022, https://tinyurl.com/32rjee52. Accessed on 13 March 2024.

[46]Mehta, Jubin, 'SHUT Clinic: An Internet De-addiction Centre Right in the Heart of Bangalore', *YourStory*, 13 April 2015, https://tinyurl.com/2y537e4x. Accessed on 13 March 2024.

Teenage and Youth

While practically all of us face the risk of developing Internet addiction, dependence is found more commonly among teenagers and early adults (15–20 years old). As per my clinical observations, people between the ages of 13 and 25, 40 and 50 (experiencing midlife crisis), and geriatric loners are more commonly affected.

The age of initiation matters. In nuclear families, toddlers are handed smartphones just so they stop crying or eat food without a fuss, or to allow parents some 'we-time', and get habituated to smartphone usage early. Schools are also increasingly using Internet-based platforms for academics. In fact, they switched to online education for long periods during the pandemic, which created the possibility of dependence for many. The only saving grace is that adolescents who go online largely for educational purposes are less likely to develop dependence.

Earlier, music, literature, arts and sports were the preferred means of self-expression. Now, many resort to creating an 'ideal self' online to overcome their self-limitations. Introverted and impulsive teenagers with underdeveloped interpersonal skills, low self-esteem and time to spare are more prone to dependence. The stressors can be related to one's academic, professional, interpersonal or family life.

Teenagers are more vulnerable for they lack the skills to process the information absorbed, and are reluctant to confide in parents lest their access to the smartphone is curtailed. Online, they get the recognition that they otherwise desire from family and friends. This acts as positive reinforcement, extending smartphone use.

It has been observed that children who mostly communicate via social media are unable to develop proper social etiquette or read the facial expressions of people in real life. They experience difficulty in forming and maintaining relationships, which has its own long-term consequences.

The online content and activities chosen demonstrate an individual's profile. Anxious people prefer gaming to overcome their loneliness through faceless socialization. Through cyber-relationships, socially awkward people manage to have total control over their image projection, tailoring their personas to get accepted without being judged. Porn addiction is thought to result from body-image problems and an avoidance of live interactions, and it can make the individual feel guilty as well.

Online existence is fraught with risks such as cyberbullying (in the form of threats, abuse or hacking) through social media platforms. It affects the fragile self-esteem of teenagers, bringing before them the demons they have been trying to escape. By sharing personal details online, unaware teenagers become fair game for unscrupulous elements.

Parents need to become cyber-literate and role models themselves so that when they give smartphones and other gadgets to their children, they can lay down what kind of usage is acceptable and what is not. Easier said than done, for teenagers argue that online existence is the new normal, and having privacy is integral to it. A compromise can be achieved, with parents and children agreeing upon the duration of Internet usage, websites visited, or mobile applications used. If worrisome usage persists, then a firm curtailment of the medium is important.

Make an inventory of Internet activities in order of

importance and time spent on each. The lowest ranked can be omitted. Pre-set alarms can prevent overuse. Reasonable goals help achieve long-term success. If the moderate approach fails, then total abstinence for some time can be enforced, to be followed by supervised use.

To help the child cope with the stress of withdrawal, irritability and sleeplessness, prepare a creative regimen of chores turned into interesting, fun activities that emphasize togetherness and promote social interaction, and encourage children to have real rather than virtual friends. Make it a point to praise and reward each effort. By restricting their own screen time, family members can be good role models. Spending time with children reaps rich dividends.

Common Consequences

Internet dependence can have many negative medical and socio-occupational consequences, leading to accumulated stress.

Physically, a person may experience carpal tunnel syndrome, spine deformities causing posture problems, giddiness, backache, eye strain, dry eyes, vision difficulties and headaches. Other consequences may be either poor eating or over-eating, which can lead to malnutrition or obesity. Obesity may in turn lead to diabetes and hypertension.

Regular breaks and stretching exercises help, but some bodily issues like vision problems and spinal changes are irreversible, causing a spiral of self-blame and guilt. Psychologically, overindulgence can lead to depression and anxiety, and vice versa. It can also cause mood swings, restlessness, rage, fatigue, dizziness, sleep disturbances, lower self-esteem, loss of attention, concentration and coordination problems, and memory disturbances. To know where you stand, assess yourself on the various scales freely available online or by simply answering 'yes or no' to the four Cs: craving, control, compulsion and consequences experienced.

Being consumed by one's online existence can lead to the neglect of family responsibilities and play havoc with marital life and relationships. Constant exposure to online outpourings of happy relationships may create dissatisfaction with one's real relationships. The term 'cyber widow' describes the plight of women who are 'phubbed', or ignored, by their partners who prefer the smartphone. Cyber-relationships and cyber-sex too can strain the marital bond. Neglected partners may become emotionally distant and seek comfort outside the marriage.

One's relationship with colleagues at work also suffers due to Internet dependence. Dependence results in reduced productivity due to avoidance or postponement of work, and may lead to job loss.

Psychiatric disorders, whether affecting primary sufferers of dependence or secondary sufferers like family members, need to be adequately treated. Comprehending the difference between use and dependence becomes an uphill task. Once a person overcomes denial, the detoxification process can start, either with a complete withdrawal or through slow taper.

Withdrawal during digital detox can create unbearable irritability and panic, hence the need for professional help. Post-detox, the task of re-establishing social contacts and occupational status takes effort, for the emotional gap with friends and family is not easy to bridge.

Counselling (family and interpersonal therapy) is the cornerstone of successful therapy. During family therapy, the idea is to blame the act, not the actor. Realizing and talking about the precursors and consequences of dependence is essential for course correction. With the family's support, a person can responsibly resume online activities—in moderation and under supervision. Total abstinence is not a practical goal. Apps can help monitor mobile usage and suggest self-help strategies. The danger of relapsing during stressful times is always there, so one needs to guard against it and seek help for mitigating stress.

Mishaps

Exploring different worlds on the Internet 'highway' can be a heady experience, but prolonged exposure to all kinds of information and trivia means no rest for the brain. This can lead to brain fogging, affecting cognitive abilities. According to studies, excessive screen use by preschool children is associated with lower white matter in the brain area linked to language and literacy skills.[47] Moreover, the absorption of all kinds of information or trivia may give a person a false sense of superiority, leading to argumentativeness.

Overindulgence in information can be problematic. In a world where fake news poses a real danger to societal peace, acting on inauthentic information without confirming the facts can have damaging consequences. Recent years have witnessed many instances of mob violence based on false information going viral online. Many people also give up

---

[47]Hutton, John S., et al., 'Associations between Screen-Based Media Use and Brain White Matter Integrity in Preschool-Aged Children', *JAMA Pediatrics*, Vol. 174, No. 1, 2020, https://tinyurl.com/ycy4vwbn. Accessed on 13 March 2024.

treatment for their serious illnesses to opt for unresearched alternatives they have found online, choosing emotion over logic.

Accepting risky challenges and clicking selfies doing dangerous activities is another online fad that can result in self-harm, as can aping negative behaviour seen on social media or gaming sites. One should be careful to not let the desire for fame on social media compromise one's safety. Intimate photos or videos shared online also become a source of anxiety if the relationship sours.

Lastly, on the Internet there is always the chance of getting caught out by digital financial frauds. The build-up of stress from all this can lead to self-harm.

A few commonsensical suggestions: if any sensitive information comes your way through social media, search the Internet to check for authenticity from multiple sources. Exit online groups spreading misinformation, or counter them with facts. Check with experts in the case of health-related posts. Before agreeing to a risky online challenge or giving out sensitive personal information or photos, think whether doing so is essential to your life. Finally, extortion should be immediately reported to elders and authorities.

Certain common traits of Internet addiction on the smartphone have emerged:

- Ringxiety—hearing the ringtone when the cell phone is silent
- Nomophobia—'no mobile' phobia, restlessness caused by the fear of losing or not having a mobile
- Digital amnesia—a tendency to not remember digitally accessible information. Problematic for students as it prevents the brain from processing information

- Google effect—a tendency to forget/not remember information that can be found through search engines

Try these tips for shrugging off your screen dependence:

- Turn off notifications.
- Turn off your phone before going to sleep, or put it on airplane or do-not-disturb mode.
- Rather than using the smartphone alarm, buy an actual alarm clock.
- Wear a watch so you don't need to check the phone for the time of day.
- Use time-management skills.
- Do not charge devices in the bedroom.
- Use pre-set alarms to monitor your time on various apps.
- Try a self-imposed ban on Internet access for some time, increasing the duration intermittently or on holidays.
- Use a browser rather than apps for social media access.
- Delete all unused or little-used apps.
- Reply to messages at fixed times during the day.
- While at work, keep the phone out of sight.
- Use techniques for recognizing and controlling problematic impulses like distraction.
- Make unlocking inconvenient by using an annoyingly long password.
- Tell your family and friends about your decision and ask for their support.

The phone may be smart, but we need to be smarter. It is important to realize that the freedom we crave online can turn into digital enslavement if we are not careful.

Acknowledgements

This book would not have been possible without the continued blessings of the Almighty.

In addition, I want to acknowledge and thank some very special people.

My Guruji, Shyam Sunder Sharma, who inspired, encouraged and persuaded me to write this book.

My mother, Chanderkanta Mehta, who has been a constant source of motivation. Her advice has mattered very much at every step of my life.

My wife, Dr Sonal Mehta, and my daughter, Devisha (Goonj) Mehta, who have been unbelievably understanding and supportive during the entire time I spent writing this book.

My editors, Dibakar Ghosh and Gauri Chopra, and my publisher, Rupa Publications, who backed me in every possible way during the entire publishing process.

www.ingramcontent.com/pod-product-compliance
Lightning Source LLC
Chambersburg PA
CBHW020232170426
43201CB00007B/401